A BELLEVUE LITERARY PRESS PATHOGRAPHY

Keep Out of Reach of Children

Reye's Syndrome, Aspirin, and the Politics of Public Health

A BELLEVUE LITERARY PRESS PATHOGRAPHY

Keep Out of Reach of Children

Reye's Syndrome, Aspirin, and the Politics of Public Health

Mark A. Largent

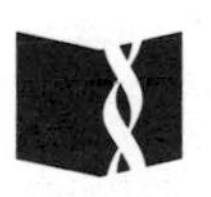

BELLEVUE LITERARY PRESS
NEW YORK

THE BLP PATHOGRAPHIES SERIES

Keep Out of Reach of Children: Reye's Syndrome, Aspirin, and the Politics of Public Health by Mark A. Largent continues the Bellevue Literary Press Pathographies series, each volume of which charts the impact of disease on human individuals and populations from the biological, historical, and cultural perspectives.

This series is dedicated to the memory of Lewis Thomas, author of several critically acclaimed books of popular science including *The Lives of a Cell: Notes of a Biology Watcher* and *The Fragile Species*. His longtime association with the New York University School of Medicine, beginning in the 1950s, influenced and inspired generations of young physicians, some of whom went on to become writers.

First published in the United States in 2015 by
Bellevue Literary Press, New York

For information, contact:
Bellevue Literary Press
NYU School of Medicine
550 First Avenue
OBV A612
New York, NY 10016

Library of Congress Cataloging-in-Publication Data
is available from the publisher upon request.

Bellevue Literary Press would like to thank all our generous donors—individuals and foundations—for their support.

Book design and composition by Mulberry Tree Press, Inc.

Manufactured in the United States of America.
First Edition

1 3 5 7 9 8 6 4 2

paperback ISBN: 978-1-934137-88-8
ebook ISBN: 978-1-934137-89-5

Dedicated with love and affection to my mom, Elizabeth Largent—
thank you for always being there for me

Contents

Keep Out of Reach of Children

Reye's Syndrome, Aspirin, and the Politics of Public Health

Prologue

In March 1972, when I was two and half years old, I contracted Reye's syndrome. I nearly died. Years later, with tears in her eyes, my mother described to me the events of those horrible days. My father was on a business trip somewhere in the South, while she and I were visiting my grandparents in Lawrenceville, a sparsely populated town in the far northern reaches of New York State. Late on a Saturday afternoon I developed diarrhea. That evening I began violently vomiting and continued throwing up throughout the night. By sunrise I was feverish and semiconscious. My grandmother knew the name of a pediatrician who had just started practicing in Potsdam, twenty miles away. Early that Sunday morning my mother called the doctor, who met us at her office.

My mother—who had worked as a registered nurse until I was born—carried me, limp and barely conscious, into the doctor's office, where she was told what she already knew: I was severely dehydrated and very ill. The pediatrician said that I had what she called a "rare condition" about which doctors knew little. There was nothing she could do for me. My mother had seen her fair share of hopeless cases in her years as a hospital nurse, and she remembers thinking that there was *always* something that could be tried. "His best chance," the pediatrician said, "is at the hospital in Ogdensburg. A doctor there has had some success with this illness." My uncle and aunt met us at the pediatrician's office in a new Chrysler my uncle had borrowed from his father's dealership. We raced forty miles west to Ogdensburg, where hospital emergency room staff had been alerted by a phone call from the pediatrician that we were on our way.

Dr. Bernard Musselman and two nurses met us at the emergency room door. "I'll never forget him," my mother told me forty years later. Musselman had attended Hamilton College in upstate New York for two years before leaving to earn a medical degree from Queen's University in Belfast, Northern Ireland. In 1958, during his senior year in medical school, he had joined the U.S. Navy, serving until 1963, and then went to work in Ogdensburg, his hometown, as a general physician. He left in 1968 to complete a two-year pediatrics fellowship at the Mayo Clinic and then returned to Ogdensburg to open his own pediatric practice. Musselman had admitting privileges at the A. Barton Hepburn Hospital, where he met us when we came racing into Ogdensburg just as church services were letting out. By then I was hallucinating and picking imaginary things out of the air.

Musselman quickly performed a venous cutdown, a minor surgical procedure that exposed the vein in my left ankle, and he inserted a line to start pumping fluids into me. That was when my mother first heard the name of the ailment that plagued me. "The doctor told me that you had a very rare condition called Reye-Johnson syndrome that no one really understood or knew how to treat," she told me later. "He said that there was a fifty-fifty chance that you would die. And, if you lived, there was a significant chance that you would have either brain or liver damage." Musselman's estimates of the prognosis for a child with Reye-Johnson syndrome—or, Reye's syndrome—were accurate, given what was known about it in the early 1970s.

It is not surprising that, despite having been a nurse throughout most of the 1960s, my mother had not heard of Reye's syndrome before my diagnosis with it in 1972. First described only nine years earlier by Dr. R. D. K. Reye, an Australian pathologist, the condition had been reported in only a handful of published cases throughout the mid-1960s. But there was little or no public knowledge of Reye's syndrome when I had it, and I was lucky that Musselman knew enough about the condition to know he must treat its symptoms as quickly as possible to give me any chance of survival. I was fortunate indeed to have been handed to a pediatrician with Musselman's rare combination of experiences: five years as a Navy doctor, which provided him with emergency training, followed by a two-year fellowship at the Mayo Clinic, one of the few places where he could have had the opportunity to learn about Reye's syndrome during the 1960s. Perhaps most importantly, Musselman knew what not to do. Throughout most of the 1960s the mortality rate from Reye's syndrome was about 80 percent, in part because physicians treated it aggressively with antibiotics, steroids, and insulin. Later research demonstrated that these early treatments were at best ineffective and at worst increased mortality rates.

Musselman ordered nurses to take blood tests every two hours and push fluids, potassium, dextrose, and glucose into me through the IV in my ankle. Despite their efforts, I grew increasingly unresponsive and fell into a coma that afternoon. My mother sat by my hospital bed through the night, and my father chartered a small private plane to fly him directly into the little Ogdensburg airport. The next day my condition stabilized. By the third day I was awake, and the IV was removed while I sipped Pedialyte and ate a sloppy joe. On the fourth day after my admission, I was released, apparently healthy and free of the brain and liver damage that half of the survivors of Reye's syndrome suffered.

Today, all that remains of my bout with Reye's syndrome is a two-inch-long scar on my left ankle, the mark of the IV line that helped save my life. There is a much deeper scar in my mother's memory of those terrifying days when I very nearly died and her worry, after I regained consciousness, about the long-term consequences of having Reye's syndrome. We did not know then that I was among the 5 percent to 10 percent of children who developed Reye's syndrome without having a prodromal illness—that is, a less serious illness that comes before the onset of life threatening symptoms. Most cases of Reye's syndrome are preceded by relatively common childhood illnesses, like influenza or chicken pox.

At the time, there was no official recording of cases of Reye's syndrome, nor was there a widely accepted set of criteria for physicians to use to diagnose it as they tried to treat it. Throughout the 1960s and into the early 1970s, Reye's syndrome was usually confirmed at autopsy, when the victim was found to have suffered the strange combination of encephalitis, the technical term for swelling of the brain, and an accumulation of fat in the internal organs, especially the liver. The symptoms of encephalitis had long been known to include headache, fever, vomiting, confusion, and loss of consciousness. In the early 1970s, Reye's syndrome's other feature—fatty degeneration of the liver—was diagnosable only at autopsy or with a liver biopsy. Because of his training at the Mayo Clinic, given my symptoms, Musselman would have suspected Reye's syndrome. He also would have known that there was no reason to bother with a liver biopsy because there was no treatment for Reye's syndrome that had been shown to be successful. A positive diagnosis would have done nothing to change Musselman's plan for treating me. All he could do was treat my symptoms and hope that I would recover.

Therapies for patients with Reye's syndrome slowly emerged throughout the 1970s; many of them were dramatic and accompanied by a host of risks. Doctors tried transfusions and total blood exchanges, they put children into drug-induced comas and used cooling blankets to force their bodies into hypothermia. To relieve pressure on the brain they removed pieces of children's skulls. Within a few years after I was hospitalized, increased public awareness and the development of less invasive diagnostic tests allowed doctors to identify Reye's syndrome earlier in its progression and to begin treatments before their patients' symptoms grew so serious that successful interventions were impossible. By the mid-1970s, physicians were ordering blood tests to check for elevated ammonia levels and indications of liver dysfunction to diagnose Reye's syndrome accurately without the need for a liver biopsy.

I was precisely the sort of child that seemed most likely to contract Reye's syndrome. Later research showed that most of the reported cases were in children who were white, middle class, and lived in the Great Lakes region, usually in rural environments. We eventually came to learn that the youngest victims of Reye's syndrome were disproportionately black and urban, but newspaper reports of the syndrome that appeared in the mid- and late 1970s were dominated by stories of middle-class white children who suddenly died with the rare combination of swollen brains and fatty livers. Their race and socioeconomic class were important factors in drawing media attention to the illness and in encouraging politicians and researchers to pay attention to it. Throughout the history of Reye's syndrome, stories about young children destroyed by a mysterious and apparently unpreventable illness haunted the pages of newspapers and professional medical journals alike. It took nearly a quarter century for us to figure out how to diagnose and treat Reye's syndrome. But before we knew what caused it, Reye's syndrome disappeared.

Two groups of researchers—a team of Australian physicians and a team of American public health professionals—simultaneously published the first descriptions of Reye's syndrome, or RS, in 1963. The illness usually begins with diarrhea and vomiting, which are followed by lethargy, weakness in the arms and legs, difficulty breathing, coma, and often death. The thousands of children who died from RS typically succumbed to respiratory distress or multiple organ failure. The unique combination of symptoms—encephalitis and liver dysfunction—seems to have first appeared sometime in the mid-twentieth century, but more than a decade passed before it was described in the medical literature. Treatment for it evolved slowly over the 1960s and 1970s. Suddenly, at the end of the 1980s, it simply disappeared. When I contracted RS in the early 1970s, Musselman was correct in his estimate of my prognosis: nearly half of the afflicted children died from symptoms associated with Reye's syndrome, and those who survived frequently suffered severe brain or liver damage from their encounter with RS.

In the early 1980s, physicians and researchers had found evidence suggesting that Reye's syndrome was much more likely to occur in children who had been given aspirin during their prodromal illnesses. From the start, aspirin had been among the many suspected factors involved in the onset of the syndrome. In the United States, aspirin was by far the over-the-counter drug most commonly given to children suffering from minor illnesses. Aspirin reduced fever, worked well as a pain reliever, was inexpensive, and had a decades-long history of safety. Its widespread use made it difficult to accept that it might be involved in causing Reye's syndrome. But the definitive cause or causes of RS remained elusive, and so aspirin stayed on the list of possible factors in the 1970s. This was in no small part because throughout the 1960s and much of the 1970s it was difficult to find children who had not received aspirin when they had minor childhood illnesses. That meant that the researchers lacked a control group of children who were not given aspirin to compare with children who had received aspirin to see if there were differences in the rates at which they developed the symptoms of Reye's syndrome.

Quite suddenly, beginning in 1980, several small research teams—all under the supervision of the Epidemic Intelligence Service (EIS) at what was then called the Center for Disease Control (CDC)—presented evidence that strongly suggested an association between aspirin and Reye's syndrome. A study of a small outbreak of Reye's syndrome in Arizona along with two multiyear studies in Ohio and Michigan produced evidence that suggested a link. A second, follow-up study in Michigan reinforced researchers' belief that there was a relationship between aspirin and the onset of symptoms associated with Reye's syndrome. Then, amazingly, as they narrowed their focus to aspirin over the next several years, the syndrome disappeared. It had peaked in 1980 with 555 reported cases; in 1987 there were only 36. A decade later, only two cases were reported. Today, cases of Reye's syndrome are rarely reported to authorities in the United States.

The medical mystery of Reye's syndrome beautifully demonstrates the challenges researchers and physicians face in identifying an unknown ailment, developing successful treatments for it, and uncovering its cause. The story unfolded over the course of two decades and involved physicians, researchers, and patients around the world. By the late 1970s, nearly every authority on the subject believed that RS was most likely a set of ailments with a number of different causes—probably several for each ailment—all of which presented with similar symptoms. A few years later, when aspirin emerged as one of the possible factors in the onset of the symptoms of RS, it seemed prudent to recommend that parents avoid giving aspirin to children who had viral illnesses because there appeared to be a correlation between aspirin and the illness.

Then Reye's syndrome became a topic for politicians, lawyers, and judges, and everything changed. The complex picture that had been slowly sketched over the previous two decades was redrawn as a caricature, and aspirin was depicted as *the* cause of Reye's syndrome. In 1982, a set of congressional hearings lambasted public health officials for scaring parents away from aspirin. Two and a half years later, another congressional hearing did just the opposite, as congressmen attacked officials from the Food and Drug Administration (FDA) and the Department of Health and Human Services (HHS) for not warning parents and doctors quickly enough to stop giving aspirin to children. The years between the two congressional hearings witnessed a spate of lawsuits over aspirin and Reye's syndrome. As the lawyers and politicians debated one another, Reye's syndrome quietly disappeared.

Lately the story of Reye's syndrome has become useful as an example in contemporary political debates. Claims have emerged asserting that pharmaceutical companies actively prevented the government from labeling aspirin bottles to protect their bottom lines, regardless of the effect on children's health. Among the most recent—and the most forceful—in making such assertions is David Michaels, an epidemiologist at George Washington University. He began his *Doubt Is Their Product: How Industry's Assault on Science Threatens Your Health*, published in 2008, with the story of Reye's syndrome, claiming that "an untold number of children died or were disabled while the aspirin manufacturers delayed the FDA's regulation by arguing that the science establishing the aspirin link was incomplete, uncertain, and unclear." The story serves as his introduction to the concept of "manufacturing uncertainty," which he describes as an increasingly popular strategy employed by individual companies or entire industries to prevent or postpone "the regulation of hazardous products by questioning the science that reveals the hazards in the first place." That strategy had, by the early 1980s, already been "successfully employed by decades by polluters and producers of hazardous products." In the case of the alleged links between Reye's syndrome and aspirin, he wrote, "The medical community knew of the danger," but the pharmaceutical industry had successfully lobbied to prevent labeling and therefore "parents were kept in the dark."

Clearly, many public health officials and epidemiologists in the early 1980s would have agreed with Michaels's assertion that aspirin was likely involved in causing Reye's syndrome, but at the time many practicing physicians did not. At the first congressional hearing in 1982, George Johnson, one of the codiscoverers of Reye's, testified that "there is nothing to this business of aspirin and Reye's syndrome . . . I have yet to talk to one of my conferees in pediatrics that does not agree." Moreover, in evaluating accusations that industry efforts slowed the process to label aspirin bottles, one should keep in mind that scientific and regulatory institutions are inherently slow, methodical animals. Salicylic acid, the active ingredient in aspirin, had been used since the time of the ancients to relieve pain and cool fevers, and aspirin had been a staple in the American medicine cabinet for nearly a century. Viewed in this light, the FDA's 1986 order that all aspirin products be labeled to warn of the potential link with Reye's syndrome came relatively quickly. Even with the supposed confirmation of the causal link between RS and aspirin that emerged with the rapid decline of the syndrome after 1980, some physicians still firmly believed that the warning came too quickly. We have, they lamented, prematurely adopted an explanation before we identified the real cause of Reye's syndrome.

Perhaps the biggest mystery surrounding Reye's syndrome is its disappearance. The ailment began appearing in hospitals in the 1950s and in the medical literature in the early 1960s. In 1980, the year that the hypothesis that aspirin might be involved in the onset of Reye's syndrome was suggested, the number of reported cases of RS peaked in the United States at 555. It is reasonable to think that there might have been years in the previous three decades that had actually witnessed more cases of RS than did 1980 because the ailment's relative obscurity led to a substantial underreporting of cases. Either way, after 1980 the annual number of reported cases fell off pretty quickly. By the mid-1990s it was very rare, and today it is almost unheard of.

The first scientifically supported claim for a cause of Reye's syndrome had emerged in the 1970s among a group of researchers and physicians in Canada. By interviewing the parents of a handful of children who had contracted Reye's syndrome, and with evidence gleaned from laboratory studies on mice, they generated evidence that implicated pesticide spraying as the cause of RS. Beginning in the 1950s, the U.S. and Canadian governments had overseen the spraying of millions of gallons of pesticides on forests to control insect outbreaks. A group of researchers led by John Crocker at Dalhousie University described how the various components of pesticides could interact with common viruses to produce the symptoms of Reye's syndrome in some children. Their claims meshed nicely with environmentalists' assertions about the dangers of aerial spraying, but met significant resistance from government officials and forestry representatives, who were concerned about the economic effects of curtailing the spraying program. Ultimately, two different scientific committees judged the Crocker research inconclusive, leading government officials to decide that the group's findings were insufficient justification to stop the spraying. But for a variety of other reasons, spraying was curtailed and the components of the spray were changed in the late 1970s, right on the eve of the rapid decline of Reye's syndrome.

Without directly arguing against Crocker's work, advocates of the aspirin hypothesis assert that the rapid disappearance of Reye's syndrome was due to warnings about a possible link between aspirin and RS that started in 1980. They claim that pediatricians and parents quickly stopped administering aspirin to children after evidence emerged of a correlation between aspirin and Reye's syndrome. Their arguments certainly seem plausible, and there is significant evidence that in fact aspirin use did decline along with reported cases of RS. This debate is part of a broader set of assertions about how careful research, expert recommendations, and a collaborative public that was committed to preventing dangerous diseases could make us all healthier and safer. As a 1999 editorial in *Pediatrics* demonstrated, by the end of the century the American public health community was trumpeting the near elimination of Reye's syndrome as "a public health triumph" and a model for "the elimination of other diseases, by means of both existing interventions and those yet to be discovered."

Later, near the turn of the century, an argument emerged that the demise of Reye's syndrome was actually caused by the recognition and treatment of a handful of inborn metabolic disorders, such as a urea cycle defect or medium-chain acyl-CoA dehydrogenase disorder. American babies born after the early 1980s—when Reye's syndrome began to rapidly disappear—were increasingly being screened as newborns for these kinds of disorders. Advocates of the aspirin hypothesis eventually accepted that at least some children with metabolic disorders were mistakenly diagnosed with RS, but they continued to assert that

Reye's syndrome was a distinct disease entity that had all but disappeared because of decreasing aspirin use in children.

The certainty that eventually developed around the aspirin hypothesis was only partly due to scientific research. The influence of the political and legal process elevated researchers' and physicians' findings to a level of certainty that the science itself could not produce. As a result, a complicated scientific question about Reye's syndrome was narrowly reinterpreted as, "What is *the* cause of Reye's syndrome?" When I spoke with Michael Thaler, a physician who had published a dozen articles on Reye's syndrome between 1970 and 1983, he explained how in the early 1980s the intensely interesting research question about the possible causes of Reye's syndrome ossified into a model that, as RS disappeared, was untestable.

As the number of reported cases of Reye's syndrome fell to near zero, a conspiracy of convenience emerged around the aspirin hypothesis. In the months and years that followed the first published reports of the studies in Arizona, Ohio, and Michigan, and the widespread media coverage of the deaths of children from RS, several U.S. congressmen developed an interest in Reye's syndrome and its alleged link to aspirin. Between 1982 and 1985, two well-publicized congressional hearings on the issue demonstrated that government officials were keen to demonstrate that they had adequately responded to the problem. In 1986, after much hand-wringing, legal action, and political bluster, the government made an agreement with pharmaceutical companies on a voluntary labeling plan for aspirin bottles. That labeling was soon found to be insufficient because it did not actually mention Reye's syndrome by name, and it was replaced a few months later by a much more robust warning to be placed on all aspirin bottles: "WARNING: Children and teenagers should not use this medicine for chicken pox or flu symptoms before a doctor is consulted about Reye syndrome, a rare but serious illness." By then, the number of reported cases of Reye's syndrome had fallen considerably, and by the time labeled bottles filled grocery store and pharmacy shelves, RS had almost completely disappeared.

But there are a number of loose ends for which the aspirin-caused-Reye's-syndrome story does not account. Cases of RS declined much more quickly than did the use of aspirin. Moreover, cases of Reye's syndrome appeared in places where aspirin was very rarely used, like Australia, and disappeared there even without a corresponding decline in aspirin use. Additionally, it appears that a number of children who never received aspirin nonetheless developed Reye's syndrome. So, at best, it appears that aspirin could have been just one of the factors in the development of the symptoms of Reye's syndrome.

Other authors, such as George Johnson, have argued that a "disease comet" caused Reye's syndrome. That is, they believed that RS was caused by a particular strain of influenza that circulated for a few decades and then disappeared. The predominance of influenza B as the identified prodromal illness in the majority of cases provided some support for this assertion, as did the rapid disappearance of Reye's syndrome in the 1980s and 1990s. But the findings from the Arizona, Ohio, and Michigan studies in the early 1980s, as well as subsequent studies by the U.S. Public Health Service, demonstrated that aspirin use strongly correlated with Reye's syndrome. It seems reasonable that some combination of aspirin use and a virus or viruses might have triggered RS.

James Orlowski, a Cleveland pediatrician in the 1980s who now practices in Florida, has long argued that the aspirin hypothesis is problematic, and he has amassed evidence to discredit it. In 1988, he published the cleverly titled "A Catch in the Reye" in *Pediatrics,* in which he demonstrated how Reye's syndrome was disappearing in Australia despite no significant change in the use of aspirin in children. Orlowski's critique of the aspirin hypothesis has met with considerable criticism. It is especially problematic to the triumphalist elimination-of-Reye's-syndrome-despite-opposition-from-industry story, which has become useful in discussions about topics like climate change or the political activities of pharmaceutical and tobacco companies.

When I started this project, I was surprised to find that there was not a single scholarly or popular analysis of the scientific and political debates over aspirin's relationship to Reye's syndrome. The closest thing I could find was an unpublished study that was available online and offered a forceful narrative about the fight to start labeling aspirin bottles with warnings about Reye's syndrome. Peter Lurie and Sidney Wolfe's "Aspirin and Reye's Syndrome" was intended to be a chapter in a textbook titled *Paradigms for Change: A Public Health Textbook for Medical, Dental, Pharmacy, and Nursing Students* that was never published. Wolfe was the cofounder and the longtime director of the Public Citizen's Health Research Group (HRG) since its founding in 1971, and Lurie was his deputy director from 1998 to 2009.

Lurie and Wolfe's analysis of the political debate over labeling aspirin opened with an emotive story—perhaps fictional, as there are no citations to support it—of a five-year-old girl with chicken pox. When her symptoms appeared early on a Saturday morning, her parents called their family doctor. The authors wrote "Take two aspirins," he said, "and call me on Monday morning." The girl developed the symptoms associated with Reye's syndrome and was dead by Tuesday night. Lurie and Wolfe reported the high mortality and disability rates that were associated with RS and referenced an article on chicken pox and aspirin published before Reye's and Johnson's 1963 papers to assert, "The etiology of the disease remains unknown but reports of its association with the use of aspirin began to surface as early as 1962, although the association had not then been demonstrated in well-designed studies." Then, in less then a page, they presented a brief summary of the Arizona, Ohio, and Michigan studies, leaving the reader with the impression that by 1981 the evidence solidly implicated aspirin as the cause of Reye's syndrome. The authors claimed that by 1984, "[t]he scientific conclusions were irrefutable: the CDC characterized the data as depicting a 'strong association between the Reye syndrome and the use of aspirin.'" The remainder of Lurie and Wolfe's chapter told of the HRG's efforts to buck the aspirin industry's intransigence and the group's ultimate victory in getting aspirin bottles labeled to warn parents of the dangers of Reye's syndrome.

For Wolfe, the account of HRG's battle to label aspirin bottles was autobiographical, because as its director he played a substantial role the story. On the heels of the CDC's initial warning about a possible link between aspirin and RS, Wolfe and the HRG released press statements, petitioned government officials, filed lawsuits, and conducted a letter-writing campaign to television and radio stations before the "final outcome of HRG's efforts was achieved on March 7, 1986 when the FDA published its Final Rule, requiring that all aspirin products have mandatory labels." Sadly, the authors concluded, it had come more than "four years and 150 deaths due to Reye syndrome after the first CDC recommendations." In their assessment, "hundreds of children had died or become brain-damaged in the interim while the government and the Executive Board of the AAP [American Association of Pediatrics] bent over backwards for industry."

The issues at hand in the early 1980s were much more complicated and far more informative of broader issues and concerns than anything that has been portrayed by its participants. This is why historians are loath to allow subjects—especially the winners—to write their own histories. We all comprehend the world through the lens of our experiences and framed by our objectives, so even the most balanced firsthand accounts are rife with assumptions, inaccuracies, and prejudices that undermine their ability to help us understand historical events in accurate and useful ways. It is a short walk from personal descriptions of history to outright justifications of the outcomes of past events. Distance from the physicians and researchers as well as genuine empathy for them and their patients gives good historical analyses the ability to inform us about past events while at the same time illuminating more general trends. The history of Reye's syndrome is full of particulars, but they are worth recounting and analyzing only if they can bring to light something bigger than themselves.

The history of Reye's syndrome reveals the difficulty Americans have enacting policy in the shadow of uncertainty. It also demonstrates how much more difficult the task is when there are competing interests at stake, even when there is a significant consensus and an earnest desire to err on the side of caution. Over the course of more than two decades, physicians, researchers, government officials, and parents struggled to do what was best for children. However, while they may have shared similar goals, they had tremendously different assumptions about the best ways to achieve them, and they followed fundamentally different paths.

This is a story of the fierce competition among different scientific and medical disciplines to prove their mettle by discovering the cause of Reye's syndrome and thus preventing deaths and devastating disabilities from a childhood disease. It reveals how deeply threatening a few scientific dissenters can be to a relatively delicate consensus about how to prevent an illness that is still not fully understood. Reye's syndrome demonstrated how quickly we made tremendous progress in reducing childhood deaths over the course of the twentieth century and how vigilant we became in preventing them. The ailment was the impetus for dozens of grassroots parent organizations that eventually merged into one organization, the National Reye's Syndrome Foundation. It was formed in 1973, and continues to educate parents and physicians about the early signs of RS and why children should never be given aspirin. Finally, in the twenty-first century, Reye's syndrome has become a textbook example of how industry representatives exploit and cultivate scientific uncertainty to prevent federal authorities from regulating their products.

Reye's syndrome has never been systematically chronicled, nor have its storytellers been carefully questioned. When we look at its story closely, we find that it is richly informative about how science, medicine, and politics interact. This book is an attempt to understand how Reye's syndrome emerged, how it was investigated, and—perhaps most significantly—how it continues to influence the politics of science and medicine long after it has disappeared.

CHAPTER ONE

The Discovery of Reye's Syndrome

It seems that every story about Reye's syndrome starts in one of two ways: either with a child stricken with the ailment—as I began this book—or with Ralph Douglas Kenneth Reye. Born, reared, and educated in Australia, Reye was the child of German immigrants. He attended medical school at Sydney University and married Corrie Saunders, a medical school classmate and later a pediatrician who specialized in the rehabilitation of children with cerebral palsy. Reye spent his entire career at the Royal Alexandra Hospital for Children in Sydney, eventually becoming director of the hospital's Institute of Pathology. In addition to describing the syndrome that bears his name, he was the first to identify fibrous hamartomas (very rare, benign, soft-tissue tumors in young children), and he was the first to describe nemaline myopathy (a congenital hereditary disorder that causes muscle weakness). "A tall, quiet, reserved man," Reye was noted for his skills as a physician and for his knowledge of Australian literature and art. He loved discussing motorcars and would happily spend "hours discussing the relative merits of car engines." A colleague who memorialized him remembered that "a highly polished, meticulously maintained, vintage white Jaguar automobile was his pride and joy." He died on July 16, 1977, a day after his mandatory retirement, of a ruptured aortic aneurysm.

Throughout the 1950s, a handful of children had arrived at the Royal Alexandra Hospital with a strange combination of symptoms. They had been recovering from flu-like illnesses but then were attacked by violent vomiting, convulsions, coma, and usually death. Many of the children had abnormally low blood-sugar levels, and their lab results indicated that most of them had severe liver dysfunction. They all showed signs of encephalitis, and every one of these children died despite every therapeutic effort. As the hospital's head of pathology, Reye had overseen the autopsies of the children, and he noted that their livers were engorged with fat, but saw no evidence of inflammation or the death of liver cells that would have suggested an infection. He also noted that the children had significant swelling of the brain, which suggested they might have been exposed to a toxin of some sort.

Beginning in 1951 and continuing throughout the decade, one or two children a year presented at the hospital with similar symptoms. By 1958, Reye had defined a set of clinical and laboratory indicators that corresponded to the findings at autopsy that he was regularly seeing. A year later, one of his colleagues jokingly wrote in a chart that the patient suffered from "Dr. Reye's Syndrome" and that Reye should therefore be consulted. What started as a joke soon became the norm, and "Dr. Reye's Syndrome" or "Douglas Reye Syndrome" was a term commonly used in the Royal Alexandra Hospital in the early 1960s to describe the ailment of children who presented with evidence of encephalitis and liver dysfunction.

Reye was a notably reserved person, and he appeared uninterested in publishing a description of the disorder that locally had been attached to his name. Two of his colleagues—Graeme Morgan, the hospital's chief resident medial officer, and James Baral, the resident pathologist at the hospital—encouraged Reye to publish. Morgan remembers approaching Reye and saying, "Listen, it's about time we reported this, and I am willing to help." With Reye's consent and advice, Morgan and Baral pulled the charts for every suspected case over the previous twelve years, finding a total of twenty-one children with remarkably similar symptoms. They also enlisted the local health department to begin investigating the homes of the children that presented with the combined symptoms of encephalitis and liver dysfunction. The product of Morgan and Baral's work was a 1963 *Lancet* paper coauthored with Reye.

The children described by Reye and his colleagues ranged in age from five months to eight years. Two-thirds of them were girls, and two-thirds were two years or under. The authors reported that all the children had experienced an "initial period of malaise" followed by a cough, sore throat, earache, and a stuffy nose. Remarkably, considering the fact that most of the children would soon die, in the early stages none of them had suffered from anything more than a mild childhood illness. After a few days—at most a week—there was an abrupt change that usually began with severe vomiting before the victims grew confused and frequently fell into comas. About half of the twenty-one children developed "wild delirium," with screaming, intense irritability, and violent movements. The other afflicted children were very restless before they slipped into comas. Almost all of the children were comatose by the time they were brought to the hospital. Seventeen of the twenty-one children suffered from seizures, and many of them experienced spasms that made their backs arch violently. Most had a characteristic posture, with flexed elbows, extended legs, and clenched hands, and all of them had been diagnosed with inflammation of the brain.

Encephalitis causes flu-like symptoms of fever and headache and, as the swelling grows more severe, patients develop confusion, seizures, hallucinations, weakness, coma, and death. The condition is recognized as an indication of an underlying problem. So when a patient presents with it, clinicians begin the process of ruling out the many different possible causes of brain swelling. Today, the most commonly diagnosed causes of encephalitis are viruses, bacteria, parasites, toxins, and fungi. In coming to a diagnosis to explain the cause of a patient's encephalitis, physicians began by excluding various possible causes starting with the most likely ones, using brain-imaging technology, spinal taps, laboratory tests, and brain biopsies to search for indicators of infection or exposure to toxic substances. When none of the known causes of brain swelling can be found, the diagnosis is idiopathic encephalitis, or encephalitis of unknown etiology. The significant contribution that Reye and his colleagues made to medicine was their recognition that at least some of the cases of idiopathic encephalitis shared the additional symptom of fatty liver. Their finding, augmented by later researchers' contributions, suggested that their patients' encephalopathies—that is, their manifestations of brain disorder—might be caused by a yet to be understood (and potentially treatable) disease or infection.

The first of the cases that Reye and his coauthors described had been admitted to the hospital in 1951, and his symptoms had led the doctors to think that he suffered from inflammation of the brain. The autopsy found no evidence of any infection that would explain his encephalopathy, and the physicians concluded that it was a unique case after they failed to find any patients who had presented in the preceding ten years with similar symptoms. Two years passed before the second patient suffering from a similarly unexplainable case of encephalitis appeared. At autopsy Reye performed a toxicological examination in hopes of identifying a poison that might have caused the child's death. He found nothing. Throughout the 1950s, as additional cases emerged, Reye came to believe that he might be dealing with a disease that had not yet been described. Some of the symptoms—especially those related to the seizures that many of the children suffered—suggested that tetanus might be the cause. But, as with the toxicological exams, no evidence was found to support that diagnosis.

When the seventh patient with similar symptoms arrived at the hospital, Reye contacted the Institute of Child Health in Sydney, which sent medical officers to the homes of all seven children. They took detailed histories of illnesses in the families, studied the children's home environments, and searched for evidence that the children might have been in contact with drugs or poisons that could explain their symptoms. In the early 1960s, shortly before Reye, Morgan, and Baral's paper was to be published, a similar study was undertaken by the New South Wales Department of Public Health. They searched for evidence that the children might have ingested or inhaled carbon tetrachloride or trichloroethylene (toxic chemicals that were used in a variety of household and industrial applications) or the insecticides dinitrate cresol or dinitrate orthocresol. At the time, these substances were beginning to raise concerns among some researchers about their potential to impair health. "This survey," the authors reported, "like the first, failed to provide any evidence of access to any likely poison or to show any relation to concurrent illness in parents or siblings." They also asserted that the search for a single cause might be in vain, as they themselves were not "entirely convinced that the ætiology is identical in every case." That is, a number of different and unrelated factors might have been causing very similar constellations of symptoms among the children they treated.

Vomiting was the one constant that all of the children experienced. In every child, the onset of violent vomiting marked the shift from a minor childhood illness to a life-threatening ailment. About half of the children eventually vomited black or dark-brown material—later authors described this as "coffee ground vomitus"—indicating that the children had blood in their stomachs. The vomiting usually subsided only as they fell into comas, and their comas almost always led to death. By the time enough children had been admitted to the Royal Alexandra Hospital for Children to warrant a report of their shared symptoms, doctors at the hospital "had become familiar with the condition."

The matter-of-fact descriptions offered by Reye, Graham, and Baral of the children's illnesses mask the horror and pain that must have been suffered by the children and their families. Routine childhood ailments had literally overnight become life-threatening illnesses as the children grew confused and antagonistic, vomited, and screamed before falling into comas. Most of these children suffered violent, unexpected, unexplainable, and devastatingly sad deaths. A decade later, when newspaper reports about Reye's syndrome began appearing in the United States, they frequently focused on the ailment's rapid onset, its unexplainable origins, and the misery it brought to the families visited by it. Throughout the 1950s and 1960s, about 80 percent of the children stricken with Reye's syndrome died, and about half of the relatively few children who survived had significant brain or liver damage. It was not until the early 1970s that the death rate from Reye's dipped below 50 percent. The families of children in whom Reye's syndrome was diagnosed were usually left with dead or badly damaged children but few answers about the origins of the devastating illness that shattered their children's lives.

The doctors were every bit as confused about the positive outcomes of Reye's syndrome as they were about the origins of the disease. Of the twenty-one children that Reye and his colleagues described, only four survived. Like the others, they had received various combinations of glucose solutions, steroids, and insulin, but they had overcome the malady and most of the other children had not. There was no apparent explanation for why some lived, and the situation was made even more confusing because many of the surviving children quickly returned to health and remained healthy thereafter. My mother frequently describes how quickly I emerged from a coma and requested something to eat. I found a report in a nursing journal in the 1970s that describes a case in which a comatose child with RS who was receiving an exchange transfusion suddenly regained consciousness and began talking.

Reye and his colleagues' 1963 article was augmented by an editorial in the same issue of the *Lancet* discussing the "new syndrome." The editors lamented, "New syndromes are always challenging." After briefly summarizing reports of the twenty-one cases offered in the original article, the editorial emphasized how little clinicians knew about the cause of the children's illnesses. Every clue that had been pursued led nowhere, every therapeutic intervention seemed equally ineffective, and the small number of surviving children had unexplainably overcome their symptoms. It seemed obvious to the editors that "some ingested poison still seems the most probable explanation" because the children's symptoms "all suggest a potent toxic agent." Just as Reye, Graham, and Baral had pointed toward analogous ailments with known causes, the editors concluded by describing the "nearest approximation to the new syndrome" of which they knew, the condition described as veno-occlusive disease, seen in children in the West Indies. That condition is "almost certainly brought about by some toxic agent in the bush teas," further suggesting that a toxin was causing the new syndrome. But, as with the physicians' attempts to isolate a bacterial or viral cause of their patients' encephalitis and fatty livers, their efforts to identify a toxin that could explain their illnesses were in vain.

Johnson's "Encephalitis-Like Disease"

While Baral and Morgan were combing through old case files from the Royal Alexandra Hospital, halfway around the world another physician was also hot on the case.

In the spring of 1962, George Magnus Johnson was assigned to investigate a handful of deaths in North Carolina that shared several troubling characteristics. Johnson was a recent medical school graduate who had joined the Epidemic Intelligence Service of what was then called the U.S. Communicable Disease Center (which was later renamed the Center for Disease Control and today is called the Centers for Disease Control and Prevention). The EIS was created in 1951, "an age when intense controversy raged among physicians, epidemiologists, and the military over biological warfare." Because of the secrecy associated with the subject, officials believed it would be "prudent to mount a major program of recruiting and training epidemiologists and to establish the closest possible bonds of respect and communication with state and local health authorities." During the 1950s and 1960s, as the draft remained in effect, many physicians participated in the EIS program as a way of fulfilling their Selective Service obligations. The EIS is still in operation, and today, as then, it is a two-year program in which students are placed in the field to provide service while learning on the job. The program emphasizes the development of epidemiologic judgment, "the reasoning process that indicates when they have sufficient data on which to make public health decisions." EIS officers are matched with assignments based on their training and interests, most of them at the CDC headquarters in Atlanta, Georgia. About a quarter of them are assigned to state or local health departments and work under the supervision of local epidemiologists. In 1962, Johnson was one of about three dozen EIS officers. After he had completed a pediatric residency in Duluth, Minnesota, he joined the CDC's Epidemic Intelligence Service and was posted to the State Board of Health in Raleigh, North Carolina.

Early in 1962, Johnson was assigned to investigate a rash of deaths from encephalitis in several different parts of the state. Over the previous two weeks, ten separate reports had been submitted to the North Carolina State Board of Health of children who had died of encephalitis of an unknown cause, and Johnson was handed the keys to a state-owned car and set loose to investigate them. Over the next three months he traveled across North Carolina, finding several more cases of encephalitis in children that could not be linked to any known cause and that included a strange fatty accumulation in the internal organs. The nature of the fatty changes to the children's livers, kidneys, and hearts were suggestive of poisoning, and at first he thought that they might have died from phosphorous poisoning. But there was no evidence that any of the children had been in contact with phosphorus, so he continued his investigations. He later recalled, "From country hospitals in the mountains, the Piedmont and the Lowlands of Carolina we gathered data, investigating each case as rapidly as possible after it was reported. None of these children survived long enough to be transferred to Duke, the University of North Carolina or Bowman Gray. Hence, no professors of pediatrics, neurology or neurosurgery became personally aware of the mysterious and deadly illness."

By April, new cases had stopped appearing, and Johnson took some time to review his findings. The deaths had started early in the year, and by spring twenty-seven children under the age of fifteen had suffered from encephalitis of unknown origin. Closer examination whittled that number down to sixteen, which was still far higher than had been seen in previous years in the state. As Johnson and his colleagues were analyzing the cases, they received a letter from the Pennsylvania Department of Health that described four deaths in children from symptoms that looked a lot like the cases that Johnson had investigated. "These children," he explained, "had a relatively mild upper respiratory disease followed by a period of apparent recovery. Three to five days later, however, there was an onset of fever, severe vomiting and hyperirritability which rapidly progressed to coma. In spite of supportive therapy, the course of each patient was described as rapidly downhill with death occurring approximately 48 hours after the onset of vomiting."

Johnson found little in the medical literature that helped him explain the sixteen cases of encephalitis with the accompanying symptoms of fatty transformation of the children's internal organs. After spending "three long and lonesome days during the middle of the investigation in the University of North Carolina medical library," with "endless inspections of *Index Medicus*, the shuffling in the card catalog, the tromping up and down the circular staircase in the back stacks and the frustrated librarian who could find so very little for me," Johnson concluded that he was dealing with an ailment that had not yet been described. Late that spring he returned to the CDC headquarters to present a twenty-minute paper on his work to a "host of critical scientists and epidemiologists at the Fulton Academy on Peachtree Street in Atlanta." He remembered "an eruption of criticism" after his talk and how flustered he was by his inability to respond to their comments. Finally, Alex Langmuir, a renowned epidemiologist, founder of the EIS, and a man who "often verbally dismembered officers who did not have strong support for their data," stood and announced, "Gentlemen, this may be of great significance. Anytime we can find more about sudden brain death in children we must do so. I commend the author of this paper."

Johnson was "buoyed by Dr. Langmuir's reaction," and returned to North Carolina to coauthor a paper with Theodore D. Scurletis, the chief of the Maternal and Child Health Section of the North Carolina Board of Health, and Norma B. Carroll, a virologist with the state laboratory. They submitted their paper to the *American Journal of Diseases of Children* in the spring of 1963, several months before Reye and his colleagues submitted their paper to the *Lancet*. That summer they heard back from the journal's editor: "It is with regret that I must inform you that the board decided to reject your paper even though they agree some of the observations are of interest and merit eventual publication. The cases occurred over a three-month period in widely disseminated parts of the state and this does not constitute an epidemic." It was, Johnson later remembered, the first rejection he had ever received from a journal. With plenty of other work to do in North Carolina and with a residency at the Mayo Clinic on the horizon, he sent the article to the *North Carolina Medical Journal*, which published it in October, the same month that Reye, Morgan, and Baral's article appeared in the much more prestigious *Lancet*.

Johnson and his colleagues began their article by describing the large numbers of children who suffered from encephalitis every year. Encephalitis can cause brain damage or death, and treatments for it typically focus on alleviating the symptoms by reducing swelling, putting the patient on a respirator to assist breathing, and administering sedatives and anticonvulsants to control seizures. They explained that in the United States about 52 percent of the 1,335 deaths by encephalitis that were recorded in 1960 were identified as "infectious encephalitis of unknown etiology"—meaning that authorities could not explain the ultimate cause of death in more than half of the people in the United States whose deaths were the result of inflammation of the brain. A year later, that percentage had increased to 56.3 percent. Most diagnosed causes of encephalitis were—and still are—caused by viral or bacterial infections. At the time, mumps and measles were the cause of about a third of the deaths from encephalitis, with chicken pox, influenza, and postvaccinal encephalitis accounting for some deaths as well. But they could not explain more than half of the deaths that occurred because of inflammation of the brain.

Not being able to identify the root cause of many cases of encephalitis was an increasingly common concern among clinicians in the early 1960s. As more and more viral and bacterial infections were avoidable with vaccines or treatable with antibiotics, lingering unexplained deaths—especially of young children—were considered more problematic than ever. Two years earlier, three researchers from Harvard—Gilles Lyon, Philip Dodge, and R. D. Adams—had described the "formidable clinical problem" clinicians faced in making a diagnosis in an infant or child who was acutely ill with fever, stupor, coma, or convulsions. "This is a condition much to be dreaded," they explained, "for it strikes without warning or follows what might otherwise be considered a relatively trivial respiratory or gastro-intestinal infection, a minor injury or operation . . . And, it may prove fatal within a few hours or days despite all known therapeutic measures; or, an even worse outcome is the subsidence of the acute symptoms leaving the patient permanently enfeebled both mentally and physically." Many of these patients' symptoms were ultimately explained as the result of viral or bacterial infections, aneurysms, kidney diseases, diabetes, toxic poisoning, metabolic disorders, or epilepsy. But a large number—as many as half—of the cases could not be explained by a specific diagnosis, leading clinicians to categorize their encephalopathies as idiopathic, meaning that their symptoms arose for no known reason. Johnson had found the article by Lyon, Dodge, and Adams during those three long days he spent in the library at the University of North Carolina, and it had encouraged him to continue investigating the cases in North Carolina.

Johnson, Scurletis, and Carroll described how the sixteen cases that they investigated were broadly distributed across the western and central parts of the state. Most of the sixteen children lived in rural areas, six were male, and all but one were white. They noted that it was "of particular interest that the peak of the cases reported coincides with that of reported influenza B" in the state, suggesting a relationship between influenza and the more serious symptoms that the children exhibited. All sixteen of the children had similarly mild illnesses before becoming much more ill, with considerable variations. Two children had complained of leg pain, six had vomited, two others had sore throats, and three of them had coughs. With the onset of symptoms of encephalitis, several of the children experienced spikes in their temperatures, and most of them had seizures and difficulty breathing. Their laboratory tests likewise showed considerable variations in spinal fluid and white-blood-cell counts. Autopsies were done on thirteen of the sixteen children who died. Every one of them had a significant accumulation of fluid in the brain, and four of the children had "marked fatty metamorphosis of the liver." Johnson noted that the livers of two of the thirteen children looked much like what was seen in cases of acute phosphorus intoxication, but toxicological studies failed to confirm that excessive exposure to phosphorus was the cause of the children's deaths. Similarly, there were no remarkable bacteriologic findings that would indicate a cause of the children's illnesses.

Johnson and his colleagues concluded with a discussion section that referenced the problems described by the three Harvard researchers who had lamented the difficulties presented by children with unexplained brain swelling. It was, they explained, a "well recognized" and a "serious perplexing problem." Like Reye and his colleagues, they pointed to some hints in the medical literature of similar cases, but by and large they found little that looked much like what they had encountered. They ended by calling on the medical community to "make every effort to identify the possible etiology" of every case of encephalitis and hoped that their report would motivate a closer examination of similar mysterious cases.

The Floodgates Open

There does not appear to be anything like Reye's syndrome in the literature prior to the 1950s, nor did the systematic evaluations that many researchers later conducted of hospital records turn up cases of the disorder before the early 1950s. Something had clearly changed by the middle of the century, and the strange combination of encephalopathy and fatty liver was suddenly common enough to elicit reports from around the world. Johnson, Reye, and their colleagues appeared to be the first to publish descriptions of the ailment, but in the years that followed it became clear that a number of other physicians and researchers were seeing similar cases at the same time. By the end of 1964, dozens of physicians published their own descriptions of cases that most certainly were diagnosable as RS. The first came from three researchers at the Royal Alexandra Hospital in Brighton, England, who reported that they had "seen at least five examples of what appears to be the same syndrome." Details of three of the cases had been presented at a conference in 1962 and later published in the *Postgraduate Medical Journal*. Autopsies of the children had found that they had severe swelling of the brain along with livers that were extremely fatty. Comparing their cases to those described by Reye, Morgan, and Baral, the English researchers concluded, "There is no doubt in our mind that the three cases shown as part of a clinicopathological conference at the Royal Alexandra Hospital, Brighton, belong to this syndrome."

Throughout the mid-1960s, case reports of encephalitis with fatty degeneration of the viscera quickly accumulated in medical journals. A week after the *Lancet* published the report from the Royal Alexandra Hospital in England, it published a letter from Keitha Corlett, a physician in Auckland, New Zealand. She had known of several similar cases and had treated two patients herself, cases she had described in 1961 in the *New Zealand Medical Journal*. Both children had presented with severe vomiting, had fallen into comas, and had died. Autopsies revealed that they suffered from encephalitis as well as fatty infiltration of the liver and parts of the kidneys. As with the cases described by Reye and his colleagues, Corlett was unable to confirm that the children had been exposed to toxic substances, and all virus studies were negative.

The inability to find indications of the causes of the children's encephalopathies and the concurrent findings of fatty livers would soon become a hallmark of Reye's syndrome.

Reported cases of encephalitis with fatty degeneration of the liver appeared throughout the early and mid-1960s, all referencing the 1963 article by Reye and his colleagues and ignoring Johnson's article. The November 9, 1963, issue of the *Lancet* brought a report from H. L. Utian and J. M. Wagner at the Transvaal Memorial Hospital for Children in Johannesburg, South Africa, stating that they had "encountered 16 identical cases," over the previous decade and that only two children had survived. Calling the children's ailment "white liver disease," they explained that they had delayed presenting their findings because they had not been able to determine "any explanation of the true nature of the disease," but they believed that it probably resulted from a viral infection or poisoning. Two weeks later, a researcher at the University of Edinburgh reported that he had seen "six, possibly eight, fatal cases in children which conform to the clinicopathological syndrome described by Reye et al." D. E. Price, one of the authors of an article cited by Reye and his colleagues, wrote to the *Lancet* to describe how his group, like Reye's, had failed to find any evidence of toxins in the children's bodies that might explain their illnesses. By the end of 1965, physicians and researchers in Scotland, Czechoslovakia, and the United States also published descriptions of similar cases they had recently seen, and Reye's syndrome had established itself firmly in the medical literature.

By the mid-1960s, the only thing about Reye's syndrome that physicians knew for certain was that it existed. They did not know how to successfully treat it. They did not know how to predict if a child would survive it. And, perhaps most important, they did not know what caused it. It would take nearly two decades before answers to many of these questions would begin to emerge. But before they did, Reye's syndrome began quickly disappearing.

What caused hundreds—perhaps thousands—of children to die every year from the relatively rarely seen combination of encephalitis and fatty degeneration of the viscera? By the late 1960s, it was obvious that Reye's syndrome was a legitimate clinicopathological entity. But it was unclear if Reye's syndrome was a new disorder or merely a newly recognized one. Before the advent of antibiotics in the 1940s and of several new vaccines in the 1950s and 1960s, childhood illnesses and death were common. It would have been easy for a relatively rare disorder like Reye's syndrome to hide among the noise of all those other illnesses.

Nonetheless, there was little in the medical literature before 1963 that resembled the ailment that would eventually be called Reye's syndrome. Reye, Morgan, and Baral had concluded their report by offering everything they could find, including a handful of earlier reports of similar cases and suggestions of analogous illnesses. They described how, a year and a half earlier, three physicians in England and the United States had published a report of the death of an eight-year-old boy who had died in Britain of an illness that sounded very much like what Reye's group had described. Physicians and public health authorities searched for evidence of food poisoning at the boy's school as well as potential exposure to fertilizers. They tried to identify sources that might have led to metal poisoning as well as cases of communicable liver disease that might explain his condition. All investigations had proven fruitless, just as they had for Reye's group.

Reye and his coauthors had also described a recent article by R. McD. Anderson that had appeared in the *Medical Journal of Australia* describing children who had died of encephalitis at the Royal Children's Hospital in Melbourne. Anderson's article pushed the first recorded RS-like case to 1950, a year before Reye's earliest case. He described how between 1950 and 1961, forty-eight children had presented at the hospital with unexplainable encephalitis, fifteen of whom also had fatty liver. Anderson grouped their ailments into categories of possible causes, but the autopsy findings of fatty liver that were discovered in half of the children suggested a strong commonality with what Reye and his colleagues had found.

Johnson and his colleagues had also pointed to several previously published papers in hope of identifying cases that appeared similar to the ones they had confronted. They cited a handful of articles in medical journals throughout the late 1950s of cases in which patients had developed encephalopathy during or immediately after they had contracted influenza. At the time, researchers referred to these as cases of postinfluenzal encephalitis or influenzal encephalopathy and had concluded that there might be certain strains of influenza that induced brain swelling. But cases were rare, and physicians had been unable to determine if particular strains of influenza had infected the patients who had later developed encephalitis, which might have suggested that a particular strain of influenza was to blame. Additionally, none of the published cases of influenzal encephalitis had described evidence of liver dysfunction or fatty viscera. However, it may be that, especially in the cases of children who survived, the physicians did not look for signs of impairment in livers because they were too busy struggling to control their patients' swelling brains.

Johnson and his coauthors also cited a recently published paper by Stuart Walker and Yasuhi Togo of the University of Maryland, who had described the case of a nine-year-old boy who had been admitted to Mercy Hospital in Baltimore in the fall of 1961 with persistent vomiting and a high fever. The boy had been healthy until five days before admission, when he was sent home from school with a runny nose, sore throat, and general malaise. That evening he grew much more ill with vomiting and fever, which continued until he was taken to the hospital, where he was briefly stabilized. But his condition worsened, as his fever spiked and he fell into a stupor, lost the ability to control the left side of his body, and began having difficulty breathing. The boy was placed on a respirator and cold blankets were used to lower his body temperature. He slowly recovered over the next several days, completely regaining normal health within a week.

Walker and Togo reported that throughout the boy's illness and recovery they had investigated possible causes of their patient's life-threatening symptoms, employing many of the same approaches that Reye's and Johnson's teams had used. Blood tests had failed to reveal the presence of bacteria that might elucidate a cause, but analyses of the child's fecal matter and spinal fluid later showed that the presence of Coxsackievirus type B. Coxsackievirus type A causes hand, foot, and mouth disease, while type B produces a range of symptoms from mild stomach ailments to chest pain and difficulty breathing as well as inflammation of the spinal cord, brain, and heart. Named after the town in New York where it was first discovered by two researchers working for the New York State Department of Health in connection with an outbreak of polio in 1948, Coxsackie B sometimes mimics the symptoms of a mild case of polio. There is still no vaccine against Coxsackieviruses, nor are there any well-accepted treatments other than time and patience. Walker and Togo concluded that the boy's illness was probably the result of infection with Coxsackie B, although they failed to find any previous reports of similar symptoms in children older than infants. Nonetheless, the boy's symptoms appeared close enough to what Johnson and his colleagues had seen in their patients for them to warrant a suggestion that they might be similar cases.

Despite a careful search, neither Reye's nor Johnson's group could find anything about the ailment they had identified in the literature before the 1960s, and there were no identifiable cases before the 1950s that compared to what they had confronted. There are two possible explanations: either the syndrome did not exist before the earliest identified cases in the 1950s, or routine childhood illnesses sickened and killed so many children before the middle of the twentieth century that it was impossible to identify the rare case of Reye's syndrome amid so many other childhood deaths. The large number of unexplained cases of encephalitis suggests that it would have been easy for the relatively rare cases of Reye's syndrome to hide among the many illnesses that struck children before we got most deadly communicable diseases came under control with vaccines and antibiotics in the second half of the twentieth century.

When I looked at the published articles cited by Reye's and Johnson's groups, one feature stood out: the ailment that would eventually be recognized as Reye's syndrome was entangled with a variety of other illnesses. Many unexplained cases of encephalitis were—and still are—categorized as idiopathic. There might have been thousands of undiagnosed cases of encephalitis with fatty liver long before it was recognized as Reye's syndrome. Or, judging from the fact that we cannot find cases before the 1950s, it might be that the ailment emerged in the twentieth century. If, in fact, aspirin sometimes triggers Reye's syndrome in children with viral infections—as we started warning parents in the 1980s—then surely there were cases of it before the 1950s. If, on the other hand, Reye's syndrome emerged as a new ailment shortly before it was described in 1963, then we would have to look beyond aspirin to fully explain its cause. Either way, once Reye's syndrome had been recognized as a "clinicopathological entity" in the mid-1960s, the next tasks would be to develop ways to quickly identify cases of it and to begin searching for its cause in hope of eliminating it or at least treating it more effectively.

CHAPTER TWO

Toxins: The Obvious Cause

In the early 1970s, several researchers began pulling together the increasing numbers of reports of Reye's syndrome in hope of explaining its origin and finding a way to prevent or effectively treat it. It seemed obvious that viruses—like influenza B and varicella, which causes chicken pox—played some role in the emergence of RS, but authors were quick to state that "a direct cause and effect relationship between influenza B infection and Reye's syndrome has not been established."

In the United States, the diagnosis of Reye's syndrome seemed to cluster within certain areas in the North and Northeast. This clustering could have resulted from a number of different factors. If the root cause of RS were a viral or bacterial contagion, one would expect the cases to cluster in areas where the infectious agent found a foothold. If it were caused by any number of different environmental factors—from pollution to food-borne illnesses—one would likewise expect to see the cases confined to certain areas. However, the clustering might be an artifact of a higher state of awareness about Reye's syndrome among health-care providers and parents in certain areas. The state-by-state variations in reporting requirements for Reye's syndrome that began to emerge in the late 1970s made the illness appear much more common in states that, like Michigan, had effective reporting requirements for RS than in states that did not mandate reporting.

While one group of researchers sought clues to the origin of Reye's syndrome, others looked for the most effective ways to identify and treat RS. The most authoritative confirmation of Reye's syndrome came at autopsy or with a liver biopsy, when a child was found to have suffered the uncommon combination of fatty degeneration of the viscera and acute encephalopathy. While a child was still fighting to survive, physicians came to diagnose RS by relying on a set of accepted biochemical indications of liver dysfunction, the symptoms of encephalitis, and the absence of any indications of the myriad infections that often caused encephalitis. Well-informed physicians would have suspected Reye's syndrome in any patient that presented with pernicious vomiting and indications of brain swelling in the wake of a minor childhood illness. Blood tests would then be ordered to determine if the child's blood was slow to clot ("prolonged prothrombin time") and if the child had elevated levels of the enzymes SGOT and SGPT (serum glutamic oxaloacetic transaminase and serum glutamic pyruvic transaminase, which help the liver break down proteins) as well as higher-than-normal levels of ammonia in the blood. By the mid-1970s, these diagnostic criteria were widely recognized among clinicians, and they corresponded closely to the autopsy or liver biopsy findings.

As the diagnostic criteria for Reye's syndrome became increasingly clear in the 1970s, some researchers found in them possible clues about the origins of RS. Throughout the twentieth century and even today, when a cause for a patient's encephalitis is identified it is usually determined to be the result of a viral or bacterial infection. But the additional symptoms associated with Reye's syndrome—particularly liver damage, the rapid onset of symptoms, and the fact that only very rarely did close relatives develop the ailment—encouraged many researchers to believe that RS was caused by exposure to a toxin rather than by an infection of some sort. Reye and his colleagues had initially suspected a toxin as the cause of the symptoms from which their patients suffered, and the medical officers who had inspected the children's homes had specifically searched for drugs and poisons that might explain their illnesses. Into the 1960s, the New South Wales Department of Public Health had sent investigators to the children's homes to look for insecticides or other household poisons that might have made the children ill. All of those investigations turned up nothing.

The search for a toxin that might cause both encephalopathy and fatty liver continued throughout the 1960s and 1970s. In 1968, two researchers at the Royal Belfast Hospital in Ireland, John Glasgow and J. A. J. Ferris, reported on the death of a four-year-old girl whose illness was similar to what Reye and his colleagues had reported. Because her symptoms suggested the possibility of exposure to toxins, they undertook a detailed toxicological investigation as part of their autopsy of the girl. Analysis of her digestive tract revealed traces of paint thinners, and there were several automobile paint shops near her home. Glasgow and Ferris concluded that her death was probably the result of exposure to these toxins rather than a bacterial or viral infection. Similarly, that year a review of twenty-one cases from the period 1954–1968 at Toronto's Hospital for Sick Children concluded that Reye's syndrome had all the hallmarks of the ingestion of toxic substances. Nonetheless, the analysis of the cases, interviews with the parents of seven of the children, and analysis of the patients' medical records turned up nothing that linked the cases. The rarity of the syndrome combined with the lack of any one identifiable triggering toxin or virus led some of the researchers in the 1960s and early 1970s to throw up their hands and speculate broadly that RS was probably caused by "an overwhelming virus infection, a toxin, or combination of factors that terminate in the same clinical and pathological picture."

In the mid-1970s, additional evidence that Reye's syndrome could be the result of exposure to a toxin emerged with the case of two siblings who had developed RS years apart from each other. In 1974, researchers at Chaim Sheba Medical Center in Tel-Hashomer, Israel, reported on the case of two brothers who had repeated episodes of vomiting and liver dysfunction that ultimately led to their deaths at ages fourteen and sixteen. One brother had his first bout with RS eight years before his eventual death, the second experienced his first symptoms only a year and a half before he died. The researchers explored whether the siblings' shared environments and experiences could account for the fact that both of them contracted Reye's syndrome. They lived near a workshop at which welding and spray painting was done, and their neighborhood's air registered increased concentrations of xylol, methylisobutylactone, butanol, titanium, and zinc chromate. But the boys had not become ill simultaneously, and the family had moved to a new neighborhood in the years between the boys' deaths, so there were obvious problems with any assertion that the toxins had led to their demise. As with all the previous cases, toxins seemed like the obvious cause, but investigators failed to find sufficient corroborating evidence to support that assumption.

Jamaican Vomiting Sickness

In addition to the nature of the illness itself, researchers were encouraged to think that Reye's syndrome was caused by exposure to a toxin because of examples of similar ailments that had known toxic causes. Reye and his colleagues had concluded their paper by drawing attention to the "vomiting sickness of Jamaica," saying that it "bears certain resemblances to this fatty-degeneration syndrome." Two South African researchers—H. L. Utian and J. M. Wagner—had also suggested that Jamaican vomiting sickness might provide a clue in the search for what they had termed "white liver" disease. In a paper they published a year after Reye's paper, they described "white liver" disease as "very similar" to Jamaican vomiting sickness, "except that in the Jamaican group the cause of the disease is apparently known." Patients had made the mistake of consuming unripe fruit from the ackee tree, which is native to tropical West Africa and was introduced to Jamaica in the late eighteenth century. Ackee fruit is a major component of Caribbean cuisine, but is dangerous when it is consumed before the fruit matures because of the presence of the toxin hypoglycin A. When it is ingested, hypoglycin A metabolizes to produce methylenecyclopropylacetic acid (MCPA), which inhibits the body's ability to oxidize certain fatty acids. As a result, fatty acids accumulate in the liver and blood-sugar levels plummet. Typically, patients suffering from Jamaican vomiting sickness experience abdominal pains a few hours after eating unripe ackee fruit and then begin vomiting. Death follows dehydration, seizures, and coma. Young children are especially susceptible to Jamaican vomiting sickness, and death is much more common in children than adults.

Case reports of people who became ill after eating unripe ackee fruit had appeared in the literature from the late nineteenth century through the mid-twentieth century, with a significant outbreak in 1954 of 151 cases and fifty-two deaths near Montego Bay, Jamaica. That same year, three researchers at the University College of the West Indies in Jamaica isolated hypoglycin A and B from the seeds and seed coverings of ackee fruit. It was not until 1976, however, that a confirmation of the cause of Jamaican vomiting sickness was published. Three researchers demonstrated that ingestion of hypoglycin A by laboratory rats led to symptoms identical to those of Jamaican vomiting sickness.

For several years in the mid-1970s, a number of authors suggested that the research conducted on Jamaican vomiting sickness might provide insight into Reye's syndrome. In 1975, two researchers at the University of Colorado Medical Center speculated that the similarities between RS and Jamaican vomiting sickness "suggested a common pathophysiology." In the midst of the hunt for the cause of Reye's syndrome, Kay Tanaka, the lead author on the 1976 report that finally identified hypoglycin A in unripe ackee fruit as the cause of Jamaican vomiting sickness, rejected the assertion that the two disorders might share a cause. In a *New England Journal of Medicine* article, Tanaka and two colleagues disputed claims made by "some pediatricians in Jamaica" who suspected that Jamaican vomiting sickness was actually Reye's syndrome. The basis for such claims rested in the many similarities the two ailments shared, including "acute onset, short course, severe vomiting, deep disturbance of consciousness and a peculiar type of fatty infiltration." However, Tanaka and his colleagues compared urine samples taken from patients with Jamaican vomiting sickness with those of children with Reye's syndrome and found that the medium-chain dicarboxylic acids and short-chain fatty acids that characterized Jamaican vomiting sickness were not found in the Reye's syndrome patients. "Thus," they concluded, "the Jamaican vomiting sickness and Reye's syndrome seen in the United States are of different causes."

Other physicians, however, believed that the research done on Jamaican vomiting sickness might provide at least some new insight into the causes of Reye's syndrome. In a letter to the editor of the *New England Journal of Medicine* that responded to Tanaka's article, several researchers asserted that the two ailments' clinical and biochemical similarities might be the "consequence of the common elevation in the concentrations of short-chain acids," and would therefore help elucidate the cause of Reye's syndrome. Tanaka responded, saying that in fact "the specific mechanisms underlying the short-chain fatty acid accumulation in these two diseases are different," and that the "mechanisms in Reye's syndrome are probably more complex." Nonetheless, speculation that Jamaican vomiting sickness might help solve the mystery of RS continued into the 1980s, with case reports that suggested "that some cases of Reye's syndrome in infants are due to causes similar to that involved in Jamaican vomiting sickness, that is, organic acid chemical toxins related to metabolites of hypoglycin."

To most of the physicians and researchers involved in the hunt for the cause of Reye's syndrome in the 1970s, its similarities to Jamaican vomiting sickness seemed to be little more than a distraction. While many of the symptoms were the same, at root something never before seen must have been happening with the children who developed Reye's syndrome. The fact that apparently every child that contracted RS had been recovering from a minor childhood illness when they had developed the symptoms of Reye's syndrome made any similarities between Jamaican vomiting sickness and RS seem moot. There was no prodromal illness in the people who contracted Jamaican vomiting sickness, nor was there any reason to expect that there needed to be one, given the fact that its cause was known.

Another issue that prevented most researchers from accepting the possibility of a similarity between Reye's syndrome and Jamaican vomiting sickness was that cases of RS appeared to occur throughout the world. Every corner of the globe—from the United States to Australia, Eastern Europe to South Africa—reported cases of it. For a toxin to be involved in causing Reye's syndrome, it would have to have been present in the many places that children developed RS. In 1966, three years after Reye and his colleagues published their paper in the *Lancet*, a researcher first suggested a possible cause that might fit this description: aflatoxins.

Aflatoxins

In 1966, the same year that authors first began using the term "Reye's syndrome" to describe the mysterious disorder that combined encephalopathy and fatty viscera, D. M. O. Becroft, a pathologist at Princess Mary Hospital for Children in Auckland, New Zealand, published a description of nine children in Auckland who had died with similar symptoms between 1959 and 1965. His cases looked very much like what so many other clinicians had reported seeing—trivial illnesses that suddenly turned deadly with violent vomiting, coma, and death. Becroft explained that the children's autopsies showed that they all had uniformly bright-yellow fatty livers and severe brain swelling. He had been in contact with Reye regarding the cases and the two men agreed that the children's symptoms and the autopsy findings matched what Reye had seen in his cases.

In discussing the possible origin of his patients' illnesses, Becroft suggested two sources that could explain the symptoms from which they all suffered: infections and toxins. Initially, on the basis of their encephalitis, many of the patients had been given a diagnosis of septicemia, which is a viral or bacterial infection of the bloodstream. However, Becroft was unable to find a common viral or bacterial infection that explained his patients' symptoms, and he concluded that infection therefore could not account for the children's ailments and that they were not dealing with a bacteria or virus that had yet been identified.

The condition of the children's livers strongly suggested to Becroft that their symptoms were caused by exposure to a toxin. It was known that many chemicals could produce fatty changes in the liver, so accidental "poisoning was one of the first possibilities suggested by the liver pathology," Becroft reported, "and is still considered likely." As for infections, he could find "no obvious history of exposure to toxins in early cases, and investigation of later cases has also been unrewarding." Another possible avenue of exposure to toxins could have been from unintentional poisoning by contaminated food. Researchers elsewhere had recently reported that many foods had low levels of aflatoxins, naturally occurring fungi that were toxic. "There has been speculation," Becroft explained, "on the possible effects on man of aflatoxins and toxic products of other fungi which many contaminate cereals." Over the next decade, Becroft's call for "epidemiological studies to investigate apparently innocuous foods as potential sources of toxins" would be met with a sustained investigation into the possibility that aflatoxins might explain the emergence of Reye's syndrome.

Aflatoxins had been first identified and described in 1960 after an outbreak of Turkey X, a disease that caused the death of more than 100,000 turkeys and ducks in the United Kingdom. Researchers determined that strains of the fungus *Aspergillus flavus*, which were found in certain groundnut and corn meals, produced the liver-damaging aflatoxins B_1 and G_1. It was soon determined that young animals were much more susceptible to the toxic effects of aflatoxins than were their more mature counterparts. This was particularly disconcerting given the fact that "groundnut meal has been recommended for malnourished children," which led Becroft to suggest that aflatoxins might account for the symptoms—especially those related to liver damage—that he and Reye has seen in their patients. Throughout the later 1960s, other researchers adopted Becroft's suggestion that aflatoxins might cause Reye's syndrome. In 1968, two years after Becroft published his hypothesis, three Canadian researchers published a report of ten children who had died of the symptoms that were associated with Reye's syndrome at the Ottawa Civic Hospital between 1952 and 1967. All had suffered from the characteristic fatty liver and encephalopathy, and their physicians had been unable to explain the source of their illnesses. The researchers concluded by explaining, "aflatoxins and the toxic products of fungi can contaminate cereals and in experimental animals have produced a severe fatty metamorphosis of the liver."

By far the most exhaustive analysis of Becroft's aflatoxin hypothesis came from a group of Thai and American military researchers in Bangkok, Thailand. Throughout the late 1960s and early 1970s, a group based at the Udorn Provincial Hospital and the South East Asian Treaty Organization (SEATO) Medical Research Laboratory in Thailand studied "Udorn encephalitis," which begins with the sudden onset of convulsions and coma and usually leads to death within a few days. The researchers found that Udorn encephalitis was similar to Reye's syndrome, and they concluded, "There can be no doubt that the disease which we have encountered in Udorn is the same as that described by Reye et al." The ailment appeared to be quite common in northern Thailand; the researchers had identified 139 cases of it in 1967 and 1968 at the main hospital in Udorn province. It had a "striking seasonal variation," with the majority of cases occurring during the rainy season at the end of the year, and it was much more common among children who lived in rural, rice-farming areas. The afflicted children's symptoms, laboratory results, and autopsy findings bore out the researchers' assertions that Udorn encephalitis and Reye's syndrome were probably the same thing.

As had Reye and the dozens of other physicians and researchers who had encountered the devastating illness in their young patients, the clinicians and researchers in Thailand had sought a possible cause to explain their patients' symptoms. After an exhaustive search, they concluded that "available data seem to eliminate all causes except toxins and viral infections." They offered several arguments in favor of a viral cause, but asserted that the patients' rapid decline and the lack of other cases within the patients' families seemed to rule out viruses. More significant, they explained, no known viral disease produced the particular combination of symptoms that every one of these patients suffered. Toxins, they concluded, appeared to have a greater potential for producing the symptoms. "In our opinion," they concluded, "fungal toxins warrant very serious consideration as possible etiologic agents of Udorn Encephalopathy." In particular, they pointed to the recently discovered aflatoxins.

Over the next several years, the researchers at the SEATO Medical Research Laboratory focused increasing attention on aflatoxins as the cause of Reye's syndrome, and their published results seem very persuasive. In 1971, they released several scientific articles detailing their work. In two of these articles they explained the findings from their work with macaque monkeys, which demonstrated the capacity of aflatoxins to cause the symptoms of Reye's syndrome. They described how, in November 1968, a three-year-old boy had been admitted into the hospital with fever, vomiting, and convulsions. "After a stormy 6-hour hospital course," they reported, "the child expired." At autopsy he was found to have suffered from significant swelling of the brain and fatty metamorphosis of the liver, kidneys, and heart. Therefore, the authors concluded, the boy had died from Reye's syndrome, or Udorn encephalopathy as it was locally known. Immediately after his death, a team of researchers from the hospital visited the boy's home to interview his parents and to collect samples of everything he had eaten before the onset of his symptoms. According to the boy's mother, for the two days before he had become ill he had eaten nothing but rice. The researchers tested samples of rice from the home and found that it contained five different fungi, which they isolated and cultured. The cultured fungi were encapsulated and fed in varying amounts to two dozen macaque monkeys. The animals that received larger doses of the fungi developed severe vomiting, convulsions, and coma before dying. Autopsies of the monkeys revealed findings similar to those of children who had died of Reye's syndrome. The researchers concluded that the "striking similarities" between these research monkeys and the children who had died from Reye's syndrome "suggest that aflatoxins should be considered as a possible factor in the etiology of this children's disease in Thailand."

Encouraged by findings from their work with the macaque monkeys, the SEATO researchers continued to publish papers throughout 1971 that further explored the possibility that aflatoxins could cause Reye's syndrome. In an article published in *Food and Cosmetics Toxiocology*, they reported on their chemical analysis from the autopsy specimens from twenty-three children that had died from Reye's syndrome. They had found detectable levels of aflatoxins in all but one of the children. They had run the same tests on samples from fifteen control subjects and had detected aflatoxins in only eleven of them (69 percent), and the levels of aflatoxins appeared to be considerably lower in the control subjects than they were in the children that had died of Reye's syndrome.

Having already shown with animal models that aflatoxins could cause the symptoms of Reye's syndrome, that aflatoxins existed in the food consumed by children who had died of Reye's syndrome, and that aflatoxins were found more often and in greater amounts in children that had died of Reye's syndrome, the team published two more articles in 1971, both in high-profile journals. The first appeared in *Pediatrics* and described every case of Reye's syndrome that had appeared at the Udorn Provincial Hospital in 1969. The authors identified sixty-seven confirmed cases of Reye's syndrome and another sixteen cases of suspected Reye's syndrome, and they provided results of laboratory tests for each of them. They also identified ten different named ailments—including Jamaican vomiting sickness, Jamshedpur fever, and white liver disease—that all shared the same basic features as Reye's syndrome and classified them all as "syndromes of encephalopathy and fatty degeneration of the viscera." The authors concluded with a recapitulation of the evidence that supported their hypothesis that at least some of these children had suffered from the effects of exposure to aflatoxins. Food in the region was contaminated with aflatoxins, the seasonal variation in illness corresponded with times of increased levels of aflatoxins in the food, and animal studies had shown that younger animals were more susceptible to aflatoxins than were more mature ones.

Near the end of 1971 the group published its sixth paper of the year, which posited the clearest and most assertive articulation of the hypothesis that aflatoxins could cause Reye's syndrome. It provided a detailed analysis of forty of the sixty-seven confirmed cases of Reye's syndrome that had appeared at the Udorn Provincial Hospital in 1969 and included laboratory data and autopsy and biopsy findings, as well as every bit of evidence that the researchers had gleaned from the children who had presented with the ailment. In the discussion section of the paper they reported that the children's symptoms and the test results were consistent with exposure to some sort of toxic agent. An accurate explanation of the cause of the illness would have to take into account the seasonal variation of the illness, the specific age group that was afflicted with it, the lack of other cases within families, and the relatively widespread area from which the children presented. Thus, they asserted, "In order to reconcile the clinical and pathologic findings with the epidemiologic findings . . . it is necessary to postulate a combination of two or more etiologic factors." Their proposed explanation described two "injuries": the first would cause relatively insignificant illness, but the second would induce a series of responses that eventually led to the vomiting, coma, convulsions, and death associated with Reye's syndrome. They concluded by offering their hypothesis that aflatoxins were an important part of the cause of Reye's syndrome.

Perhaps *a* Cause, But Not *the* Cause

In retrospect, it might seem odd that the SEATO researchers were not quickly recognized for their identification of the cause of Reye's syndrome. They had offered strong evidence in favor of their claim that aflatoxins were the cause of Reye's syndrome, but their work generated very little interest from the broader community of researchers who were growing interested in Reye's syndrome through the 1970s. In fact, their work seems to have been largely ignored, even though an increasingly large number of physicians, researchers, and the public turned their attention to Reye's syndrome in that same period. No one argued that Udorn encephalopathy and Reye's syndrome were not the same disease entity, and no one published criticisms of the SEATO researchers' methods or results. At best, it appears that later researchers accepted that some Thai children developed the symptoms of Reye's syndrome after ingesting food that contained aflatoxins.

The SEATO researchers themselves had been restrained in asserting that they had discovered the cause of Reye's syndrome. For example, in one article they stated, "It should be stressed that, although encephalopathy and fatty degeneration of the viscera may be the response of some children to aflatoxin poisoning, it does not necessarily follow that such toxicity is responsible for all cases of Reye's syndrome." They typically limited the significance of their findings to only children in the northeast region of Thailand. For example, one of their 1971 articles concluded, "Supporting evidence strongly suggests that the northeastern Thailand syndrome represents acute toxicity to aflatoxins, the toxin produced by certain strains of the fungus *Aspergillus flavus*." Similarly, that same year in another article they concluded that aflatoxins "may be a factor in the aetiology of [encephalopathy and fatty degeneration of the viscera] in Thailand."

I think the aflatoxins hypothesis for Reye's did not end the discussion about the source of RS because no one who advanced it actually believed that there was a single explanation for RS. It was only after the aspirin hypothesis came to dominate discussion of Reye's syndrome that the notion that there was a single cause was born. Throughout most of the 1970s, researchers would not have bothered trying to discover a single cause of Reye's syndrome; Reye himself had believed that there were probably a number of causes for the symptoms that he and his colleagues had described. The SEATO researchers had likewise always emphasized the fact that they had, at best, discovered in aflatoxins one of the causes of Reye's syndrome. This is further evidenced by the fact that they published a list of ten different "syndromes of encephalopathy and fatty degeneration of the viscera," of which Reye's syndrome was but one, and most of the others on the list had either unknown, viral, or different toxic causes.

Throughout the 1970s, the aflatoxins hypothesis was discussed only occasionally, and it was never recognized as a suitable explanation for the source of all of the increasingly large number of cases of Reye's syndrome that were being identified and reported. Nonetheless, additional evidence in support of the SEATO team's hypothesis emerged throughout the 1970s. In 1972, Becroft published a letter to the editor of the *British Medical Journal* describing his finding of aflatoxins in the organs of two children that had died from Reye's syndrome in New Zealand. That same year, a group of Czechoslovak researchers published two articles that supported the aflatoxins hypothesis. In 1976, three researchers from the Mayo Clinic reported a case in which they had discovered aflatoxins in the liver of one of eight patients with Reye's syndrome whom they had studied. Two years later, three physicians and researchers at the University of Mississippi reported that they had discovered aflatoxins in the blood of a Reye's syndrome patient.

In 1979, the University of Mississippi group published the most extensive and authoritative argument in favor of aflatoxins as a factor in Reye's syndrome. They reported on eight children who had been admitted to the University of Mississippi Medical Center in Jackson, Mississippi, over a three-and-a-half year period in the mid 1970s. They found that at least six of the eight children they studied had aflatoxins in their livers, and they presented a summary of the evidence that supported their assertion that aflatoxin B_1 "is in some way related to" Reye's syndrome. Recent research had demonstrated that young infants that contracted Reye's syndrome typically came from lower socioeconomic urban environments, while toddlers and children diagnosed with it were predominately middle class and came from rural or suburban environments. Most of the children studied by the team from the University of Mississippi were very young and came from poor families. The researchers suggested these circumstances led to a greater likelihood of encountering aflatoxins because of the nature of their living conditions and the fact that they were probably fed the same food adults ate at an earlier age than would children raised by families of higher socioeconomic status.

The mounting circumstantial evidence emerging throughout the 1970s that implicated aflatoxins as a cause of Reye's syndrome led the CDC to study the question more closely. To do this, they used a case control study, a type of retrospective observational study that is frequently used to study the patterns, causes, and effects of health issues. In case control studies, two groups of individuals with differing health conditions are identified and compared to determine if a hypothesized cause explains a health difference between the two groups. Typically, these sorts of study are used to identify factors that contribute to a medical condition by comparing a group of people who have the medical condition with a group that does not have the medical condition but are otherwise similar to the individuals who do have the condition. When the studied outcome is rare and there are few subjects that have the health condition that is being studied (as with Reye's syndrome) case control studies are often the only feasible approach.

Any question of whether or not aflatoxins were a cause—much less *the* cause—of Reye's syndrome was put to rest in 1980 with the publication of the results of the CDC's case control study. Climatic conditions in the southeastern United States in 1977 had led to unusually high levels of aflatoxins in the corn and peanut crops, providing the opportunity to study aflatoxin levels in the blood and urine of children with Reye's syndrome, members of their families, and matched control subjects. The study identified seventeen patients whose symptoms met strict criteria for a diagnosis of Reye's syndrome early in 1978, immediately following the appearance of elevated levels of aflatoxins in U.S. crops. The seventeen patients were matched with ninety-one control subjects selected from neighborhood friends of the patients, siblings, and non–Reye's syndrome patients selected from the hospitals. There were no significant differences in aflatoxin levels between the children in whom Reye's syndrome had been diagnosed and those who did not have RS. The report concluded, "The data presented in this case control study indicate that Reye's syndrome patients are not exposed to aflatoxins at a greater rate than matched control subjects."

Despite the similarities of their symptoms, neither Jamaican vomiting sickness nor aflatoxin poisoning could provide an adequate explanation for Reye's syndrome. Nonetheless, toxins remained the most obvious possible cause for RS because nothing else seemed capable of adequately explaining the fatty degeneration of the liver that became the hallmark of Reye's syndrome. In the early 1970s, another explanation for the cause of Reye's syndrome emerged from the work of Rachel Carson, the American marine biologist who is credited with helping to initiate the modern environmental movement.

CHAPTER THREE

The Deadly Mist

IN 1962, A YEAR BEFORE Reye and Johnson published their accounts of an apparently new childhood illness, Rachel Carson's *Silent Spring* had raised public alarm about the dangerous effects of chemicals in the environment. Carson documented the devastating effects of the widespread use of pesticides on the environment, and her work helped lead to the banning of DDT in the United States. In *Silent Spring*, Carson synthesized data and case studies that were already well known within the scientific community into a format that was accessible by the general public. She offered stark conclusions about the impact of pesticides on wildlife, plants, and people. Fifty years later, her book and her subsequent efforts as a citizen-scientist are widely recognized to have spawned the modern environmental movement by awakening a new era of environmental consciousness.

In addition to sounding alarms about environmental degradation, *Silent Spring* increased fears among both the public and health professionals that new illnesses—like Reye's syndrome—might be caused by the growing number of environmental pollutants. These concerns were furthered in the 1970s as researchers began to develop evidence showing that exposure to chemicals could increase the potency of viruses in laboratory animals. Motivated by increasing numbers of children presenting with Reye's syndrome, attention turned to the possibility that toxins might combine with one or more viruses to cause RS. Because the research had obvious implications for the safety of certain commercial products, some of the researchers who were hunting for the cause of Reye's syndrome quickly found themselves tangling with well-funded industries, frustrated by sluggish elected officials, and under threat of lawsuits.

In the early 1970s, John F. S. Crocker, a professor in the Department of Pediatrics at Dalhousie University and a physician at the Isaak Walton Killam Children's Hospital in Halifax, Nova Scotia, hypothesized that Reye's syndrome might be caused by some combination of insecticides and viruses. Crocker and his colleagues had treated several children who had been flown to their hospital from remote areas, presenting with symptoms that were identical to the cases of Reye's syndrome that had been described in the literature over the previous decade. They noted that the majority of the cases came from an area in New Brunswick that had relatively few children. "The thing that was most striking," Crocker later explained about the region from which his patients came, "was that they had had a very very aggressive forestry management program, and they sprayed liberally with chemicals." The clustering of affected children in areas that were heavily sprayed led Crocker and his colleagues to examine the known effects of the insecticides and eventually to suggest that insecticides might somehow have caused the children's symptoms.

Eventually, Crocker and his colleagues discovered that the most effective opponents of their efforts to link pesticide spraying with Reye's syndrome were not the industries that sprayed the chemicals. Instead, the stumbling block was set by the epidemiologists, who failed to corroborate the evidence that Crocker and his colleagues were developing in their labs. The province's politicians accepted the epidemiologists' findings and were thus unwilling to act without a greater degree of certainty than Crocker's work could provide.

Operation Budworm

The insecticides that Crocker and his colleagues suspected might be involved in causing Reye's syndrome were widely sprayed throughout eastern Canada to control outbreaks of spruce budworms (*Choristoneura fumiferana*). The larvae of spruce budworm emerge from their silken tents in the early months of summer to eat pine needles and buds for four to six weeks. They are tremendously destructive throughout the northern parts of North America, and the economically important balsam fir is particularly vulnerable to them. Over the course of the twentieth century, budworm outbreaks had grown increasingly more frequent and more widespread. Outbreaks appeared to occur naturally at an average interval of about thirty-five years, but human-induced changes to the forest—fire prevention, clear-cutting, and the use of pesticides—had made forests more prone to attacks. The 1910s had witnessed a moderate outbreak of spruce budworm in eastern Canada and the United States, and there had been more widespread and devastating outbreaks in the 1940s and 1950s. A massive infestation of spruce budworm between 1970 and 1975 affected more than twice as many acres of trees as had all the century's previous outbreaks.

To limit the impact of spruce budworm, in 1951 the Canadian government employed twenty Wasp Stearmans—1930s military biplanes—to spray the insecticide DDT over almost 200,000 acres of New Brunswick forest. The results appeared effective enough to warrant expansion of the program, and Operation Budworm, as they called it, became an annual event. In 1952 the Canadian government established a private corporation, Forest Protection Limited, to use surplus World War II aircraft to spray insecticides and fire retardants to protect Canadian forests from insect and fire damage. Over the course of the 1950s and 1960s, Operation Budworm grew to cover 2.6 million acres of forest, blanketing them every year with literally tons of DDT. By the 1970s, widespread aerial spraying of insecticides was a common practice throughout eastern Canada and the northeastern United States to control budworm outbreaks and protect valuable forests.

Given growing concerns over possible environmental and health impacts of the increasingly common use of chemicals, it is no surprise that some researchers began to question the unintended consequences of projects like Operation Budworm. In *Silent Spring*, Carson had described the environmental impact of DDT spraying for spruce budworm in Mirimichi, a region in northeastern New Brunswick. In a chapter titled "Rivers of Death," she told of how in the early 1950s the upsurge in spruce budworm populations had been combated with small-scale spraying, but by 1954, "the planes visited the forests of the Northwest Miramichi and white clouds of settling mist marked the crisscross pattern of their flight." The impact on life in the forest was unmistakable: "Within two days dead and dying fish, including many young salmon, were found along the banks of the stream. Brook trout also appeared among the dead fish, and along the roads and in the woods birds were dying. All the life of the stream was stilled." Originally, the planes in Operation Budworm sprayed a pound of DDT over every acre of forest. In 1954, that amount was reduced to one-half pound per acre "for purposes of economy as much as for other reasons."

DDT was used on forests in Canada and the United States until the late 1960s, when, under public pressure to find a suitable replacement, forest managers began using fenitrothion, an organophosphate that was found to be "marginally less toxic to birds, enough that it could be safely used in amounts effective against the budworm." Fenitrothion and other newly introduced organophosphates appeared to be a good substitute for DDT because laboratory studies suggested that they would break down in the environment more quickly than did DDT. By 1970, fenitrothion was being widely used in both the Canadian and the U.S. spraying programs. At the same time, the costs for spraying skyrocketed because fenitrothion was more expensive than DDT and larger outbreaks of spruce budworm required more acres to be sprayed.

By the mid-1970s, the provincial government of New Brunswick was paying most of the $20 million-a-year bill for the fleet of forty-eight airplanes that sprayed 10.5 million acres with insecticide. The lumber and pulp companies, government officials, and the people hired to spray New Brunswick's forests with fenitrothion all claimed that the spraying was necessary to protect both the province's forests and its economy. Rudy Hanusiak, the Deputy Minister of Natural Resources, declared that without spraying, 90 percent of the province's pulp mills would shut down because there would be no lumber to feed them. Even as spruce budworm attacks in New Brunswick became more frequent and more costly, the province's economy became increasingly reliant on its forest industries. At the same time, increased mechanization in the forests and the mills led to a decrease in the number of employees the industry could support, which caused pressure to maintain as high a production rate as possible. When some researchers began to question the safety of aerial spraying, the public was presented with the claim that spraying was necessary to maintain a healthy economy regardless of potential negative health effects on citizens and the environment. The New Brunswick provincial government chose to continue its efforts to maintain the health of its economy instead of reducing or eliminating spraying to avoid a potential environmental or public health disaster. "I don't like to see people dying," said New Brunswick's minister of natural resources. "This is one of the things that I really wouldn't like to see. But, as the same time, knowing the forest as it is, my decision will have to be with the forest and with the future of New Brunswick."

From the start, scientists had played a critical role in raising concerns about the unintended consequences of aerial spraying. The earliest organized opponents to spraying against spruce budworm had been a handful of sportsmen's organizations that had expressed concern over its effects on their prized game fish, the Atlantic salmon. As early as 1950, some scientists also participated in debates over aerial spraying. C. J. Kerswill and P. F. Elson, two biologists at the Atlantic Biological Station in St. Andrews, had investigated the effects of DDT spraying on Atlantic salmon. In 1955, they published reports of extremely high death rates among salmon and aquatic insects in the streams in areas that had been sprayed with DDT. Conservationists like Ott Hicks published articles in Canadian newspapers and magazines that drew from Kerswill and Elson's work to publicize claims that aerial spraying would lead to the "virtual elimination of algae and food organisms so vital to [the] well-being and growth of young fish, perhaps for years to come." Supporters of Operation Budworm, including the deputy minister of lands and mines, W. W. McCormack, angrily responded that such claims were written "in an alarmist tone" and expressed "a great many fears far in advance of scientific proof." Sportsmen's resistance to spraying faded as DDT was abandoned in favor of fenitrothion, which broke down more quickly in the environment and presumably had less of an impact on wildlife. However, a pattern in which different interest groups and their allied scientific experts contradicted one another was already established when, in the early 1970s, concerns about aerial spraying shifted from protecting the region's salmon to protecting its children.

Timmy Keddy and the Concerned Parents Group

In January 1972, a ten-year-old boy named Timmy Keddy contracted influenza, which had been running through his entire family. The Keddys lived in Durham Bridge, a small town in central New Brunswick. When Timmy began vomiting violently and his fever spiked, his parents took him to the Victoria Public Hospital in Fredericton, the provincial capital. Timmy's six-month-old sister developed similar symptoms and was also admitted to the hospital. She recuperated quickly, but Timmy's condition grew worse. The next day he fell into a coma and was flown an hour southeast to the Izaak Walton Killam Hospital for Children in Halifax, Nova Scotia. His case was taken over by John Crocker, who diagnosed Reye's syndrome. That night, Timmy died without ever regaining consciousness.

Timmy Keddy was one of at least nine children in whom Reye's syndrome was diagnosed over the previous two years at the hospital where Crocker practiced, and one of the five who had died there from RS. Crocker and several of his colleagues began investigating possible causes, and they suspected some sort of chemical poisoning. Nothing in Timmy's home could explain his illness, and his symptoms were so similar to the handful of other local cases that Crocker's team suspected an environmental contaminant rather than a household poison. They turned their attention to the chemicals that were being sprayed by Operation Budworm and hypothesized that the insecticides were the root cause of the growing numbers of diagnoses of Reye's syndrome in the area.

By the early 1970s, evidence had already emerged that exposure to insecticides, herbicides, or other chemicals might make children and other young animals much more susceptible to typically nonlethal viruses. As was the case with aflatoxin, it appeared that exposure to some of the chemicals used in commercial insecticides might be much more harmful to children than they were to adults. Unlike aflatoxin, which had no commercial use and was regarded by everyone involved as a problem, the insecticides were sprayed to protect the valuable timber that was under attack by spruce budworm. As a result, Crocker knew that any research that suggested that the spraying ought to be curtailed was likely to meet stiff resistance from the timber industry and its allies. As

Crocker later explained, "Because of the controversy about spraying, we never published the data because we felt that we would end up in court from the threats we were getting from the industries."

Despite the perceived threat of lawsuits, in 1974 Crocker and four other colleagues published a paper in the "Preliminary Communications" section of the *Lancet* that discussed their research inducing in mice the symptoms associated with Reye's syndrome by topically applying various components of insecticides to the animals, then exposing them to a virus. Previous studies had found that at least some young animals were more susceptible to death from viruses when they had been exposed to some of the components of common insecticides. To "determine if exposure of young animals to insecticides increases their susceptibility to viral infection," Crocker and his colleagues applied different combinations of two commonly used insecticides—DDT and fenitrothion—to the backs and abdomens of two-day-old mice for eleven consecutive days. Two days later, they exposed the mice to sublethal doses of the encephalomyocarditis virus. The results were striking. The control subjects, which had been rubbed with corn oil and exposed to the same virus, all survived. The mice that had been exposed to DDT had a maximum mortality rate of 8 percent, and the mortality rate for the mice that had been exposed to fenitrothion was twice that. However, the mice that had been exposed to both DDT and fenitrothion had a remarkably high mortality rate—sometimes as high as 60 percent.

Crocker's goal of identifying *a* cause—if not *the* cause—of Reye's syndrome was obvious in that first paper, and the research team focused its attention on the insecticides sprayed by Operation Budworm. In the paper's introduction, the authors stated, "Our interest was stimulated by the observation that cases of Reye's syndrome . . . occurred in children living in areas of heavy forest insecticide spraying." Likewise, in the discussion section, they described how cases of RS "seem often to happen in geographically circumscribed areas" and concluded, "the concept of exposure to insecticides or other chemicals, such as herbicides, followed by or concomitant with virus infection, as causal, is quite attractive to us." While other researchers made brief appearances in the literature exploring the connection between insecticides and Reye's syndrome, Crocker's efforts to link Reye's syndrome with insecticide spraying persisted for decades.

Even though the results of their work seemed to point to Operation Budworm as a likely cause of the cases of Reye's syndrome in their area, Crocker and his colleagues' 1974 *Lancet* article received no media attention in New Brunswick. The researchers had been cautious in presenting their early findings, and the work had been published as a "preliminary communication," highlighting its relative immaturity. To advance the research, Crocker and his colleagues needed to know precisely what was being sprayed, which turned out to be a difficult piece of information for them to obtain. Crocker later described how senior managers at the timber companies and at Forest Protection Limited had refused to provide his team with details of the ingredients of the insecticides, but the employees who were actually doing the spraying eventually gave the researchers samples of the spray. The insecticides consisted of three components: a toxin designed to kill the target pests, one or more solvents, and a blend of emulsifiers. The solvents were used to dilute and extend the toxins, and the emulsifiers acted as wetting agents to help disperse the insecticide. Without a wetting agent, Crocker explained, the insecticides would "just sit as a glob on the leaf," and emulsifiers were used "by the trainload" and in "liberal amounts."

Upon closer scrutiny and with additional experiments, Crocker's team came to believe that the emulsifiers—not the toxicants or the solvents—were most likely responsible for causing Reye's syndrome. In 1976, two years after they published the initial report of their research in the *Lancet*, they published an article in *Science* in which they reported that contact with the nontoxic components of insecticides increased the lethality of some viruses. As in their earlier work, Crocker and his colleagues painted the abdomens of day-old mice with different combinations of corn oil (as a control), DDT, fenitrothion, solvents, and emulsifiers, then exposed the mice to mouse encephalomyocarditis virus. They found that the mortality rate was much higher in the mice that were exposed to the mixture of solvents and emulsifier than it was in the controls or the animals exposed to the toxins alone. The toxic components of the spray did not substantially increase the lethality of the virus, but the solvents and emulsifiers that most authorities had considered unproblematic apparently did. Crocker and his colleagues concluded that the widespread use of pesticide dispersal agents and emulsifiers were therefore considered "safe on substantially insufficient grounds."

Crocker Goes Public

In March 1976, several months before Crocker's team published their *Science* article, a newspaper journalist in Cape Breton, Nova Scotia broke the story of a possible link between Operation Budworm and Reye's syndrome. The Nova Scotia government had recently approved a plan to spray 100,000 acres for budworm in the Cape Breton Highlands. The publicity surrounding the research and Crocker's description of the team's findings compelled authorities in Nova Scotia to hold a special session of the cabinet and invited Crocker to describe the team's conclusions. That same day, the minister of health announced that the spray program was cancelled. A week later, a story in the *New York Times* declared, "Rare Children's Disease Tied to Solvents Used in Pesticides," over a second story describing the death from Reye's syndrome of a twelve-year-old New Jersey girl. Shortly thereafter, Crocker was interviewed about his research on Canadian Broadcasting Corporation (CBC) Radio. The publicity that emerged from the stories and the interview attracted the attention of the New Brunswick provincial government, which had the nation's largest spraying program against spruce budworm.

Unlike Nova Scotia, where government officials chose to suspend spraying immediately, leaders in New Brunswick convened a committee of experts to review Crocker's research. W. G. Schneider, president of the National Research Council of Canada, chaired the panel of six medical and agricultural experts. Schneider was a physical chemist and an expert in nuclear magnetic resonance; he was also a highly respected scientist and administrator whose reputation and talents added significant authority to the committee's findings. Schneider's committee met for three days later that month, reviewed the available evidence, and heard testimony from, among others, Crocker. The committee concluded that, even though the results published by Crocker and his colleagues offered support for a link between Reye's syndrome and the spraying of insecticides, considerable uncertainty remained. It agreed that Reye's syndrome was most likely multifactorial; that is, it involved and perhaps required a number of precipitating elements. But it also found that the incidence of Reye's syndrome in New Brunswick appeared to be no greater than it was in areas that did not spray and for which statistics were available. Moreover, it discovered that cases of RS seemed to arise during times of the year when spraying did not occur. The research published by Crocker and his colleagues suggested a link, they said, but the studies needed refinement and replication by other research teams, which had not yet happened. Therefore, the committee members concluded that more research and better monitoring was needed before they were willing to accept definitive conclusions about a link between spraying and Reye's syndrome.

As the expert panel's findings were being released and the New Brunswick government was formulating a response, a grassroots movement against aerial spraying emerged to pressure government officials in New Brunswick to halt the program. The parents of two children who had contracted Reye's syndrome made a public plea to the government of New Brunswick to halt the spraying. In interviews with the CBC and other members of the Canadian press, the parents of Timmy Keddy and the parents of a nine-year-old girl who had survived a bout with Reye's syndrome called for the government to halt spraying "if there is even the slightest indication it may be linked to the rare but often fatal children's illness." Both sets of parents reported that they had lived in or frequently visited areas that had been heavily sprayed.

Given the inconclusive findings from the expert panel, the momentum in favor of spraying, and perception of the tremendous economic risk that the spruce budworm represented to the province's economy, New Brunswick's government officials chose to continue the spraying program in 1976. In making their decision, they adopted a conventional approach to risk management that required unequivocal proof of harm before changing policy or implementing new regulations. Such an approach risks overlooking damages caused by unproven threats and maintains the status quo. It also places a tremendously high burden of proof on researchers like Crocker who were attempting to alter policy with scientific evidence that suggested that the current policy might be causing harm to the environment or to public health. Often, this conventional approach to risk management establishes an impossibly high burden of proof on reformers, something that has been demonstrated again and again in issues ranging from Reye's syndrome to climate change to vaccines.

In the face of the New Brunswick government's decision to continue its massive spruce budworm spraying program, in 1976 several local citizens formed the Concerned Parents Group, which led public protests against spraying and negotiations with government officials for the next decade. They called on the government of Quebec to halt plans for a $15 million plan to spray nearly nine million acres of forest. Over the previous twenty years there had developed "a feeling of powerlessness and mistrust among some members of the general public over the way the forests were being managed." When evidence emerged that Reye's syndrome might be caused by the spraying, there had already been in place both resentment about forest policy and a sense that government officials were deaf to complaints about the spraying program.

Over the summer of 1976, opposition to spraying spread to other provinces, as parents who worried about the potential health effects of spraying began expressing opposition to Operation Budworm. As was the case with the environmentalists who had preceded them, the Concerned Parents Group had little immediate impact on public policy. New Brunswick's spraying program was intensified as authorities tried to save the province's stands of balsam fir, a common target for the spruce budworm and a natural resource that was critical to the province's economy. The spraying program grew to cover 9.2 million acres at a cost of nearly $19 million. On May 11, 1976, eleven airplanes lifted off from the Blissville Airstrip in southern New Brunswick and began the year's annual spraying of the province's forests. By the end of that summer, J. R. Bedard, a director of the Canadian Forestry Association, explained that the spraying program had been necessary because, without spray, "instead of a green forest we would've had a grey one, a tinderbox, a real mess." He declared, "We may have to spray next year, the year after that and the year after that if that's what it takes to keep the forest green."

New Brunswick's 1976 spraying program was the largest ever, covering about half of the entire province with a mist of fenitrothion. The government's refusal to halt the program on the basis of the expert panel's conclusion that there was insufficient evidence that the spray was indeed harmful was met with cheers from industry and growing resentment from some parents and environmental groups. Earlier that summer, reports emerged that government officials had been made aware of a possible link between spraying and Reye's syndrome as early as 1971, but had made no effort to inform the public of possible dangers. Near the end of the summer, the *Ottawa Journal* published a long exposé by journalist Russell Hunt titled "Biological Warfare in New Brunswick." The article began with a description of the death of Timmy Keddy, then explained John Crocker's efforts to discover its cause. Hunt explored the development of Operation Budworm, the emergence of Reye's syndrome, and Crocker's research on a possible relationship between the two. It offered a clear depiction of the stark contrasts that existed between the two sides of this issue: on the one hand were parents who appealed to the government to stop spraying in order to preserve their children's health, and on the other hand was an industry on which the entire province relied saying that the spraying was necessary to preserve the health of the forest and thus the province's economy.

Hunt's article elicited a pair of letters to the editor of the *Ottawa Journal*, both of which demonstrated the tortured and contentious nature of the issue. Carol Dumont, a mother in Windsor, Ontario, who had lost her five-year-old son to Reye's syndrome a year earlier, wrote to congratulate the paper for having the integrity to print Hunt's article. She reported that her son had died three weeks after Windsor had been sprayed. "Why," she asked, "are the legislators so callous?" A week later, L. A. Adams wrote to describe how he had read Hunt's article "with my fists clenched, my teeth gritted and my heart pounding with rage." With his anger directed at "those concerned with and in control of the budworm spraying programs," Adams asked, "What more proof do they need that it is pesticides that cause Reye's syndrome? And even if it turns out that it is not pesticides, why take the chance?"

The lack of definitive evidence supporting a causal link between aerial spraying and Reye's syndrome met with calls from scientists for increased investments in research. Additional funding did emerge, and it addressed the problem in two fundamentally different ways. In December 1976, Canada's Environment Minister Vince McClean announced a $14,000 grant to study tetradecena, a potential replacement for fenitrothion that might safely and effectively disrupt the spruce budworm's ability to reproduce. Later that month, the National Research Council of Canada released a report on *Bacillus thuringiensis* (Bt), a soil-dwelling bacterium that appeared to work well as an insecticide, and since it was naturally occurring, it might have fewer adverse effects on the environment and on human health than the synthetic insecticides might have had.

A court case involving aerial spraying demonstrated that while Crocker and his team continued their work, the industries that supported the spraying were hiring researchers to develop evidence that the spraying was safe. Abram Friesen had operated a family farm near Fredericton, New Brunswick on organic principles. During the 1976 spraying season his farm—and his family—was sprayed. Both Abram and his wife, Marie-Luise, testified that they suffered lung pains and feelings of fatigue after being sprayed while they were picking fiddleheads near a brook on their farm on May 21, 1976. They also reported that the spray caused an asthma attack in their son and killed several hundred bees and some of their livestock. In response, Forest Protection Limited produced two expert witnesses who testified that the spray had no effect on humans or the environment. Junshi Miyamoto was a senior researcher for Sumitomo Chemical Company of Osaka, Japan, the company that sold fenitrothion to the New Brunswick government. According to the *Ottawa Journal*, "He described numerous experiments, conducted by himself, that showed the pesticide was safe." The company also brought to the stand Morris Shelanski, a toxicologist who, at the request of Forest Protection Limited, had explored the effects of fenitrothion on humans. He testified that "he had done tests in which capsules of a fenitrothion solution 250 times as strong as that used in the spray program were given to human volunteers without effect." The case made its way to the New Brunswick supreme court, which decided that the government had no legal right to spray insecticide over private land. The *New York Times* reported, "Shortly thereafter, the government introduced a bill in the provincial legislature to allow private land to be sprayed without the owner's consent."

In April 1977, as the next season of spraying approached, the National Research Council of Canada funded a symposium titled "Fenitrothion: The Long-Term Effects of Its Use in Forest Ecosystems." Crocker and his colleagues' work was front and center, and they were joined by a team of researchers from Ohio State University, who described the prior work that had been done on virus–chemical interactions that demonstrated that some chemicals, such as DDT and fenitrothion, could drastically increase the potency of poliovirus, vaccinia, and the virus that caused foot-and-mouth disease. They concluded by offering a working hypothesis that "suggests a multiple etiology" for Reye's syndrome that included viruses, chemicals, or some combination of the two. Their conclusions fit nicely with the work that Crocker and his colleagues were doing, and their contributions suggested that there was growing support for the idea that investigations into the unintended effects of environmental toxins might help uncover the cause of Reye's syndrome.

A year later, Crocker was guest editor of an issue of *Chemosphere,* a British journal devoted to environmental chemistry. The issue consisted of seven original research papers—including one from the Ohio State research group—that focused on "the possibility that Reye's syndrome, an acute, potentially lethal childhood entity, may be an environmentally induced disease." Crocker was a coauthor on five of the seven articles, and he wrote the short editorial for the issue. In it, he expressed hope that "the collection of papers presented here will clarify" the issues raised by the alleged association between certain environmental chemicals and Reye's syndrome. He also noted, "The area of research enclosed in this issue . . . is potentially one of the most explosive environmental issues in the world today, and therefore should be of interest to all scientists."

Resistance to Canadian provinces' spraying programs continued to grow throughout the late 1970s as an increasingly large coalition of groups voiced concerns about possible harmful effects on the environment or on the public health. In 1978, the movement spread to nearby Newfoundland and attracted "some respectable participants to the side lined up against the government." A citizen group—People Against the Spray—formed and drew support from the Newfoundland Medical Association, the Women's Institute, and even the local branch of the Canadian Air Traffic Controllers Association. At the same time, the loggers' unions voiced support for the government's decision to continue spraying. The issue became politically polarized in Newfoundland, where Progressive Conservatives supported spraying while the province's opposition Liberals opposed it. Newspapers in eastern Canada continued to publish occasional stories of children who had contracted Reye's syndrome that frequently asserted a connection between RS and spraying. By 1979, the issue had developed to the point that television shows like *Across Canada* offered hour-long investigative reports focusing on the "controversy surrounding the link between insecticides and the deadly children's disease Reye's syndrome," and newspapers in the region published feature stories with titles like "Spray Wars! Are the Risks Worth the Results?" At the same time, the controversy over spraying and its alleged relationship to Reye's syndrome arose in discussions about spraying programs in the United States, although it never developed into as big of an issue in the United States as it did in Canada.

Throughout the late 1970s and into the 1980s, Crocker and his colleagues continued researching the links between aerial spraying and Reye's syndrome, and in 1978 they published results of their research on kidney cells from African green monkeys. Crocker and three other researchers had investigated whether cells exposed to the emulsifiers in insecticides were more easily infected with viruses than were cells that were not first exposed to emulsifiers. They examined the effect of seventeen different commercially available emulsifiers on six different viruses (vesicular stomatitis virus, encephalomyolcarditis virus, vaccinia virus, Herpesvirus type 1, reovirus type 2, and poliovirus type 1). As with their earlier work, their findings were alarming. "There is little doubt," they concluded, "that enhancement of virus infection by some emulsifiers is substantial." Moreover, the greatest level of viral enhancement occurred at concentrations that were less than toxic. So exposure to these emulsifiers at lower, presumably safer, levels actually caused viruses to infect cells as much as four times faster than they did in control subjects. Single-stranded RNA viruses—which include both influenza A and influenza B viruses, the two viruses that caused the most common prodromal illnesses in children suffering from Reye's syndrome—were enhanced by exposure to emulsifiers, while DNA viruses were not.

As the aspirin hypothesis rose to prominence in the early 1980s and the annual number of reported cases of Reye's syndrome fell to near zero by the end of the decade, Crocker and his colleagues persisted in their research exploring the possible links between RS and insecticides. Their 1980 article in *Applied and Environmental Microbiology* demonstrated that an emulsifier that had "an environmental relationship to Reye's syndrome" increased the rate of virus penetration on a culture. From that research, they concluded, "Reye's syndrome may have, as one etiological factor, an environmental intoxicant which has the capacity to compromise the interferon response," and thus the emulsifiers used in the spraying against spruce budworm may be "involved in the causation of a local outbreak of Reye's syndrome." Later research by Crocker and his colleagues continued to focus on ways in which emulsifiers retard the body's ability to combat viruses, and all of their resulting publications were directed at identifying the cause of Reye's syndrome. Their work focused almost entirely on animal research, which contrasts sharply with the epidemiological research that was employed in evaluating it. Eventually, Crocker and his colleagues' experiments involved a very large number of animals—about 42,000 in total. "These weren't just a couple of dozen animals exposed to chemicals and then exposed to human virus," Crocker later remarked.

In the early 1980s, a growing number of reports in the popular media further increased concern among Canadians about the potentially negative health effects of the spraying for spruce budworm. In 1980, the CBC aired "Poison Mist," a radio program hosted by Bert Deveaux. It offered a particularly sensationalistic presentation of the possible link between Reye's syndrome and Operation Budworm, describing fenitrothion as "a nerve gas developed during World War II" that caused cell mutation in laboratory tests. Deveaux incorrectly claimed that Reye's syndrome "struck only communities close to sprayed areas," then introduced Timmy Keddy's mother, Betty. She described Timmy's final days: "He had the flu for about two or three days. Thought it was over. Up playing around for about a day. That night he came down sick again. Sort of delirious. Took him to the hospital the next day. Before the night was over he was in a coma. Four days later he was dead." Deveaux presented Timmy's case as representative of something that was increasingly common in New Brunswick, claiming that the province "had an epidemic on its hands." In response, he said, the government "turned its back on its own advisors" by refusing to make a full study of Reye's syndrome. Deveaux's depiction of the possible link between spraying and Reye's syndrome fundamentally mischaracterized a number of issues, villianizing government officials and oversimplifying a complex set of problems. But it also demonstrated the growing fear and frustration many parents felt about the spraying programs.

As public concern about spraying continued in the early 1980s, Crocker and his colleagues stoked it with a 1982 article in the *Canadian Medical Association Journal* that showed that one of the suspect emulsifiers, Toximul MP8, caused cellular damage in laboratory mice that paralleled cellular errors identified in children with Reye's syndrome. They hypothesized that the emulsifiers prevented the normal recovery of children from some viruses by compromising the body's interferon response, a cellular response to the presence of pathogens that allows cells to communicate with one another and mount an immune response. By comparing blood samples from five children who had contracted influenza B and had then developed Reye's syndrome to samples from children with influenza B who had not devolved RS, the researchers found that the children with RS appeared to produce a far weaker interferon response. Given the laboratory findings that suggested that emulsifiers weakened the interferon response, they concluded that the chemicals "may be a significant feature in the genesis of Reye's syndrome." According to observers, the study "generated considerable concern and apprehension among persons living in areas sprayed to control spruce budworm and prompted other researchers to investigate this matter further." Newspaper reports of their findings asserted a strong connection by claiming, "tests with human tissue have verified a link between Reye's syndrome and chemical spraying." In an interview with the CBC journalist Deveaux, Crocker's coauthor Kenneth Rozee claimed that the group's findings "should remove any medical or scientific objection to stating that a clear link exists between Reye's syndrome and spray emulsifiers." Rozee concluded, "The problem is no longer a scientific one, but a political and economic one.

Enter the Epidemiologists

"Science" is often popularly described in such a way as to suggest that it operates with a single shared set of methods (typically referred to as "the scientific method") and then speaks with a single voice. "Science says . . ." is frequently hurled as an undeniable last word in a political debate and usually with more than just a hint of authoritarianism. The "science says . . ." portrayal contrasts sharply with the ways in which many scientists view their enterprise, which is typically as a massive, multidisciplinary, ever-evolving set of tools, data, approaches, and conclusions. Historians, philosophers, sociologists, and other scholars have long explored the different ways in which science is understood by scientists and by nonscientists, and they have concluded that the situation is impossibly difficult to characterize easily. Science is an enormous enterprise and it has no single voice—and no pope or monarch—who speaks for it. More important, though, are the vast differences between scientists and nonscientists in the ways in which scientific information is perceived when it is considered as part of the political process. When it becomes involved in political deliberations, the inherently democratic, deliberative, and objective nature of scientists' work contrasts sharply with the authoritarian and static depiction of science and its findings within political debates.

Health and environmental issues are particularly vulnerable to the effects of the different ways in which scientists and nonscientists perceive the usefulness of scientific research, especially when powerful financial interests are involved. In part because of the ways in which scientific evidence is wielded in political debates and in courtrooms, the public has grown wary of the capacity of science to make definitive claims about politically or economically charged issues. As far back as the 1950s—when Kerswill and Elson published their work on the effects of DDT on Atlantic salmon, Hicks drew on it to call for a halt in spraying, and the Deputy Minister of Lands and Mines called their concerns "alarmist" and offered "far in advance of scientific proof"—it was evident that scientific authority could be brought to bear on either side of the spraying issue. In his 1976 exposé, "Biological Warfare in New Brunswick," Russell Hunt accurately summarized the situation: "It is clearly an argument that goes on and on indefinitely, with each side bringing in its own battery of 'experts' and staking out its own position." To make matters worse, the ability to shape the direction of the relevant scientific research by investing in particular research agendas allowed various parties in the debate to generate scientific evidence in favor of their preferred position, as was the case when the Japanese company that made fenitrothion directed one of its senior researchers to investigate the safety of the insecticide or when Forest Protection Limited hired an independent toxicologist to determine if fenitrothion was dangerous to humans.

One of the ways in which we have tried to overcome the problems of partisan scientific research and the polarization of science is by asking nonpartisan institutions—scientific organizations, government funding agencies, universities—to convene expert panels. In 1982, Brenda Robinson, minister of health for New Brunswick, did just that when she called for the creation of a task force to explore the possible adverse health effects associated with the spraying program. The task force was headed by Walter Spitzer, chair of the Department of Epidemiology and Health at McGill University and included pediatricians and epidemiologists from the United States and Canada. The group had two objectives: to estimate the incidence of Reye's syndrome in New Brunswick over the previous decade and to investigate the alleged association between Reye's syndrome and exposure to spruce budworm spraying.

The task force flew teams of research assistants to thirty-two hospitals around New Brunswick and six others in adjacent provinces. They examined over three thousand charts and found only twelve confirmed, four possible, and seven doubtful cases of Reye's syndrome over the ten-year period. At only .50 to .67 per 100,000, the incidence rate for Reye's syndrome in New Brunswick was lower than had been previously reported in studies of RS in Ohio and Michigan. When the group compared the location and timing of cases, they found that "no geographic or temporal associations were evident between exposure to the spray used for controlling spruce budworm in New Brunswick and the occurrence of Reye's syndrome." Perhaps even more damning to Crocker and his colleagues' insecticide hypothesis for Reye's syndrome was the task force's finding that there was no difference in the number of confirmed cases of RS in the Saint Johns district of New Brunswick during a five-year period of heavy spraying as compared to the five-year period of light spraying; each showed the same number of cases despite a drastic difference in chemical exposure.

Shortly after Spitzer's New Brunswick task force completed its work, two researchers at the Maine Department of Human Services' Bureau of Health began a similar study in Maine. Robert B. Wood, Jr., and Gregory F. Bogdan compared Reye's syndrome incidence rates in towns that had been sprayed for spruce budworm infestations against those that had not. While recognizing the New Brunswick task force's conclusion that there was no evidence to suggest a connection between RS and spraying for spruce budworm, Wood and Bogdan explored the wider variety of chemicals that were used in Maine to control the insect. They obtained a list of twenty-seven cases of Reye's syndrome that occurred in Maine between January 1978 and December 1982 and produced an annual incident rate of 1.48 per 100,000, which was considerably higher than the rate calculated by the New Brunswick task force. Only one of the twenty-seven cases occurred in an area that had been sprayed for spruce budworm. Wood and Bogdan concluded, as had Spitzer and his colleagues, that their data "do not support the existence of an association with spruce budworm insecticide spraying and the increased incidence of Reye's syndrome."

Crocker and his colleagues had established, using laboratory tests, that the chemicals being sprayed on forests could make relatively benign viruses deadly. Had a correlation between spraying and Reye's syndrome existed, their work would have helped researchers establish that spraying and RS were not merely correlated, but that there was a causal relationship. However, epidemiological analyses could not identify a correlation, and without a correlation no causation could be established even if a cause was possible. So, despite its apparent capacity to explain Reye's syndrome, Crocker's insecticide hypothesis was not accepted as an explanation of the cause of RS. As the aspirin hypothesis emerged late in 1980, rhetoric about how children were being sacrificed in order to save the forest faded from public discussions about Reye's syndrome.

But Crocker's work on Reye's syndrome fundamentally advanced our understanding of the ailment by helping focus attention on the liver and away from encephalitis. By asserting a toxic cause for RS, encephalitis came to be seen as a problem that itself had been caused by liver dysfunction. Crocker's work also shows us the stark difference in approach between laboratory science and epidemiology. While Crocker focused on possible causes, the epidemiologists focused on correlations, which would ultimately prove the final arbiter in separating possible causes from actual causes. In the end, the epidemiologists influenced the political leaders to a much greater degree than did Crocker and his colleagues.

While laboratory scientists and epidemiologists were struggling to identify the cause of Reye's syndrome, physicians and other clinicians were fighting the front line battle against the illness. Over the course of the 1970s, as Reye's syndrome grew increasingly better known to clinicians and parents, physicians developed more effective ways to diagnose and treat the disorder. Their work is perhaps the most dramatic part of the story of Reye's syndrome.

CHAPTER FOUR

The Front Line in the Battle against Reye's Syndrome

SOMETIME DURING 1969, six years after Reye and Johnson published their respective papers, the professional discussions about Reye's syndrome fundamentally changed. Before 1969 there had been a number of short articles and many letters to editors from physicians who had seen patients suffering from its now familiar symptoms. By the end of the decade, that conversation had turned to identifying the typical course of RS, its possible causes, and potentially effective treatments. The medical literature reflected that shift while slow but steady progress was made against Reye's syndrome. Those same articles also demonstrated a growing frustration among many of the physicians who treated an increasing number of children afflicted with RS every year. They worked on the front lines battling Reye's syndrome, and their journal articles and public statements about RS give us a glimpse of their growing frustrations with the deadly disease they battled and the limited resources—both in terms of money and knowledge—that they had to fight it.

Perhaps the clearest indication of the shift in the nature of the professional conversation about Reye's syndrome and the undeveloped nature of physicians' understanding of the ailment came in a 1969 editorial in the *Lancet* that summarized what had been learned about it to date. To be more accurate, the editorial showed just how much was not known. The editors briefly summarized the 1963 paper by Reye, Baral, and Morgan as well as the flood of reports that followed it and the efforts to identify earlier cases and disentangle them from similar ailments. They described the characteristics that had come to be associated with Reye's syndrome and asserted that there had not yet been any recognized diagnostic blood tests that could confirm the presence of the disorder; only a liver biopsy or autopsy finding of fatty degeneration of the viscera along with encephalopathy could do that. There were, however, a number of laboratory findings that often appeared in conjunction with the symptoms of RS, such as low blood-sugar counts, blood tests that indicated liver dysfunction, reduced total carbon-dioxide content, elevated blood-urea levels, occasionally high sodium levels, and often elevated levels of ketones. But not a single one of these laboratory findings was present in every child who was diagnosed with Reye's syndrome, so they were of limited value in confirming diagnoses.

The authors of the 1969 editorial in the *Lancet* also described how researchers and physicians had been unable to determine the cause of Reye's syndrome, although several reasonable explanations had been suggested by that time. Viruses—including adenovirus type 3, Coxsackie A, reovirus, herpes simplex, echovirus and influenza B virus—had been identified in patients with diagnosed Reye's syndrome. However, as was the case with the laboratory findings, no one virus was found in most, much less all, of the patients. Some authors suggested a toxic cause for RS, while others compared it to the vomiting sickness of Jamaica or believed that at least some cases might be caused by aflatoxins in the children's food. As with laboratory tests, there was no toxicological test or finding that explained a significant number of identified cases of Reye's syndrome. The editors concluded, "Of course, no single cause may exist and this syndrome may simply represent a common reaction to a variety of stimuli, some of which may be infective or toxic."

While there was considerable uncertainly about what might cause Reye's syndrome, the physicians and researchers who published papers about it in the early 1970s had enough evidence to develop a few widely held assumptions. First, cases of Reye's syndrome seemed to cluster in certain regions while they were entirely absent in others. It would be relatively easy to explain these findings as an artifact of differences in the levels of awareness of RS from one region to another, but careful studies of case files at hospitals in regions that were free from Reye's syndrome convinced most researchers that the cases did indeed appear in some areas and not in others. The cases clustered not only in regions but also in time. There was a Reye's syndrome "season" that ran from January through March, the same months in which influenza was most common. Reye's syndrome was also rare, and most physicians would never see a case. This meant that every case deserved intense scrutiny to help researchers learn as much as possible about the uncommon ailment. Its rarity also suggested that for some reason certain children might be vulnerable while most others were not, which led to intense interest in any case in which siblings contracted RS. Finally, given the tremendous range of regional, socioeconomic, and racial factors—children from all over the world were diagnosed with Reye's syndrome—there were probably multiple causes of RS. Several authors suggested that Reye's syndrome probably represented a collection of fundamentally different illnesses that shared a similar presentation.

Advancing physicians' knowledge about Reye's syndrome, effectively treating the children who suffered from it, and ultimately eliminating it required quick and accurate diagnosis and effective treatments, both of which began to emerge in the early 1970s. Most cases in the 1960s had been confirmed with a liver biopsy or, more frequently, at autopsy. Effective early interventions required the development of less invasive diagnostic methods as well as a framework to describe the progression of the illness and identify how far a child's health had deteriorated. And physicians needed proven treatments for Reye's syndrome, and they needed to be able to develop treatments that were specific to the each stage of the illness. These tasks were clinical in nature, and thus were confined to the physicians who encountered critically ill children in the hospital. But there was hope that early identification and the development of more effective therapies would provide additional evidence for the researchers who were searching for the cause or causes of Reye's syndrome.

The Clinical Staging of Reye's Syndrome

The brutality of Reye's syndrome was fully confronted by the physicians and nurses who struggled to save individual children's lives. The relatively sterile clinical descriptions offered in medical journal articles usually masked much of the horror, uncertainty, and devastation that unfolded in patients' lives. Often the children's deaths are not even overtly announced in the articles; instead, the case description of the child's symptoms and laboratory results abruptly ends and a new section of the paper begins that describes the findings at autopsy. As the numbers of cases each year increased, the medical journal articles started to deal with general trends in presentation and treatment of Reye's syndrome and shifted away from individual case reports, which had often contained painful details about each child's condition, the damages RS inflicted, and often the child's death. As a result, the personal experiences of patients, their parents, and their health-care providers were increasingly camouflaged in the medical literature.

In contrast to the formal accounts of children battling Reye's syndrome that are found in the medical journals, far more vivid accounts of the terrible destruction RS wrought on afflicted children and their families began to emerge in the 1970s from advocacy organizations like the National Reye's Syndrome Foundation and in newspaper articles and television news accounts. Perhaps the most wrenching of all the accounts I have seen is one that was produced in 1976 by Chicago's CBS affiliate WBBN. It described some of the twenty-six cases of Reye's syndrome that were treated at the Cincinnati Children's Hospital in 1974. The grainy black-and-white film begins with the image of a child, comatose and on a ventilator. An announcer narrates, "This is the horror of Reye's syndrome. Six-year-old Denise Harden of Covington, Kentucky, unconscious now as she has been for the last six days. Despite eight blood transfusions, her condition remains critical. If she does live, her brain will be damaged forever." Another child, a seven-year-old, is shown awake and breathing on her own but clearly quite ill. Her speech is badly slurred and she is confused and obviously uncomfortable. Half of the fifty-five children treated with Reye's syndrome at Cincinnati Children's Hospital over the previous decade, the announcer tells us, died. "Early treatment is vital," he states, "but no one knows which treatment is best." The sounds and images of screaming children and distraught parents are painful reminders of the toll taken by Reye's syndrome. The doctors' frustration with their limited capacity to help them is especially obvious in the film.

The dramatic popular accounts of Reye's syndrome did much to advance the public's knowledge of the ailment and provided physicians the opportunity to see more children in the early stages of RS. Professional recognition and public awareness of the symptoms of Reye's syndrome encouraged parents to bring children suspected of suffering from RS to the hospital more quickly, allowing physicians to explore additional ways to treat the children before they developed much more dangerous symptoms. But to take advantage of the opportunity of seeing cases earlier in their progression, physicians needed an accurate framework to distinguish the different stages of Reye's syndrome and to begin to develop accurate assessment tools and effective treatments. These tools were not available until the mid-1970s, after enough cases had been carefully studied and compared in order to establish the illness's normal progression.

In 1974, a group of physicians from Boston led by Frederick Lovejoy proposed a set of guidelines for describing Reye's syndrome in various cases to help establish the relationships among and between the various symptoms that had come to be associated with RS. Called "clinical staging," the system allows physicians to describe the state of a patient's symptoms in a standardized manner and prescribe appropriate therapies for each stage. The goal of therapy would be to prevent the patient from "progressing" (which, frankly, is a strange term to use in this context since we hardly think of more serious symptoms and being closer to death as "progress") by employing treatments that have been demonstrably effective for patients at a particular stage. Clinical staging is therefore a valuable tool in both chronicling the typical course of an ailment and in treating a patient. Lovejoy and his colleagues conducted a retrospective study of forty patients with Reye's syndrome over a three-year period between 1968 and 1971 "in the hope that this could provide a basis for more logical treatment in the future." Seventeen of the patients had died and two of the survivors had severe brain damage. From the histories of forty patients, they constructed five distinct stages in Reye's syndrome, each with its own symptoms and diagnostic criteria, and they began the process of identifying appropriate therapies for each stage:

Stage I: vomiting, lethargy, sleepiness, and laboratory evidence of liver dysfunction

Stage II: disorientation, delirium, combativeness, hyperventilation, hyperactive reflexes, appropriate responses to pain, and laboratory evidence of liver dysfunction

Stage III: coma, hyperventilation, a decorticate posture (in which the patient has bent arms, clenched fists and holds his or her legs straight out), eyes react to light, and laboratory evidence of liver dysfunction

Stage IV: deepening coma, decerebrate posture (in which the patient holds his or her legs straight out with toes pointing downward and an arched back—an indication of severe damage to the brain), eyes no longer react normally to light but have large and fixed pupils, often only limited laboratory evidence of liver dysfunction

Stage V: seizures, loss of reflexes, respiratory arrest, and a generally limp posture.

American physicians quickly adopted Lovejoy's framework for the clinical staging of Reye's syndrome, and it became a valuable tool in both the treatment of Reye's syndrome and in discussions about the causes of RS. But it could only describe the typical course of the illness; it could not disentangle symptoms from the cause or causes of those symptoms, nor could it offer much direction about which symptoms to treat most aggressively and which ones to accept as corollary and thus of less importance in developing a scheme for treating patients.

Reye and his colleagues had offered little help to clinicians who looked to them for advice on how to treat children who presented with the symptoms of Reye's syndrome. They introduced their paper's short section on treatments with the disclaimer, "It cannot be proved that any form of treatment has altered the outcome"—which was death in seventeen of the twenty-one cases they described and a return to completely normal health in the other four. Because many of the children had low blood-sugar levels, they had been placed on glucose IVs. When they failed to show the expected improvement, physicians also administered steroids and sometimes insulin. The best results they were able to obtain came in the cases that received relatively high levels of glucose and hydrocortisone intravenously. Three of the four children who survived had received this treatment. Reye and his colleagues concluded, "Since we had become accustomed to regarding the outlook as almost hopeless, this has created a fairly strong impression that the treatment had some bearing on the outcome." Clearly, given the tremendous amount of uncertainty surrounding Reye's syndrome and its very high fatality rate, their standards for evaluating a therapy's effectiveness were quite low.

The SEATO researchers in Thailand had offered a similarly discouraging description of their efforts to find successful interventions. Their usual course of treatment for the ailment was large doses of antibiotics and steroids, and in the late 1960s they had begun giving the afflicted children tracheotomies and putting them on respirators in hope of helping their bodies struggle through the effects of the illness long enough to overcome it. However, they concluded emphatically and in italics, "*In no case did therapy appear to influence the course of the disease.*" Treatments for Reye's syndrome, especially the early ones, were therefore experimental—often to the point of seeming haphazard—because the ailment was so new and physicians had very little guidance. Parents were desperate, especially as Reye's syndrome became better known and feared in the 1970s, and were obviously willing to try anything that might help their children survive their brushes with the mysterious and deadly disorder.

Over the course of the 1970s, through trial and error and with hints from the treatment of analogous ailments, physicians developed treatment protocols for Reye's syndrome. One set of treatments focused on the symptoms, especially those associated with encephalitis. The growing pressure in the children's brains often caused brain damage, and most of the children that died as a result of Reye's syndrome typically died from respiratory failure caused by encephalitis. To prevent the swelling of the brain from causing irreversible brain damage and eventually death, physicians developed a number of practical ways to relieve the pressure and placed the children on mechanical respirators to keep them breathing. The second pathway along which therapies for Reye's syndrome developed attempted to address the underlying cause of patients' encephalitis, which was increasingly recognized to be the result of liver dysfunction. From the start, the unique combination of fatty degeneration of the liver and encephalopathy differentiated Reye's syndrome from other ailments that caused swelling of the brain. But it was not clear if both of its characteristic symptoms were the result of a single unrecognized cause, or if one of the identified symptoms was causing the other one. By the late 1960s, several physicians had been encouraged by research on liver disorders to think that impairment of the children's livers was leading to their encephalopathy. If that was the case, the best treatment for Reye's syndrome—and the true source of RS—was to be found in the problems that arose in the children's livers. Therefore, the therapies that emerged from this approach focused on treating their blood chemistry in hope that the children would return to health.

In both types of therapy—those that addressed encephalitis and those that addressed liver dysfunction—the physicians' goal was to help their patients weather the symptoms of Reye's syndrome long enough to overcome the ailment. As a result, by the mid-1970s patients with RS who were being treated by well-informed physicians would likely have received treatments that drew from both these therapeutic pathways as their doctors paid close attention to their symptoms and their progression through Lovejoy's five stages. Many of the children ultimately survived the effects of liver dysfunction and encephalitis without permanent damage and they returned to normal health. But many others did not.

As physicians developed therapies for Reye's syndrome, it became increasingly important for them to identify cases of RS as early as possible so that they could carefully chart the course of the children's illnesses and engage the most effective therapies at each stage. It was in this context that clinicians and advocacy groups for Reye's syndrome cooperated to spread the word about Reye's syndrome and to encourage parents and health-care providers to increase their "index of suspicion" about the syndrome. Throughout the 1970s, the mortality rate for children in whom RS was diagnosed fell from about 45 percent at the start of the decade to about 25 percent by 1980. Early diagnosis became the most important factor in the increasing success that physicians had in helping their patients survive Reye's syndrome. But, as we will eventually see, it also brought Reye's syndrome to the public's attention in a manner that led to increasingly strident calls by parents, journalists, and politicians for physicians and researchers to find the ailment's ultimate cause quickly and eliminate it.

Addressing Liver Dysfunction

While some physicians focused on the problems associated with the children's encephalitis, others considered encephalitis a by-product of liver dysfunction and focused on relieving the symptoms associated with liver failure. These treatments for Reye's syndrome drew guidance from research on hepatic coma, which followed the most severe neurologic symptoms that accompanied severe liver disease and included tremors, personality changes, and confusion. Throughout the 1960s, physicians who specialized in liver diseases had developed a number of treatments for hepatic coma, including transfusions and even dialysis. As these approaches were shown to have some success in treating patients with acute hepatitis, they were increasingly adopted by physicians to treat Reye's syndrome.

Peter R. Huttenlocher, a physician and professor of neurology at Yale University Medical Center and later at the University of Chicago, helped pioneer treatments for liver dysfunction in Reye's syndrome patients. Huttenlocher, a pediatric neurologist, was renowned for his clinical skills and quickly became an expert in Reye's syndrome in the early 1970s. After Huttenlocher's death in 2013, a colleague remembered his early interest in Reye's syndrome and his empathy for the children who suffered from it as well as for their parents. For Huttenlocher, Reye's syndrome was both a medical mystery and a terrible ailment, and he devoted a significant amount of his time and energy to finding ways to diagnose and effectively treat it.

Huttenlocher's first contribution to the medical literature on Reye's syndrome came in 1969, when he was the lead author on an article in *Pediatrics*. Along with two colleagues, he reported on ten patients with

Reye's syndrome and described their method of diagnosing RS in them without a biopsy or autopsy by using blood tests that would reveal elevated blood-ammonia levels. The presence of higher than normal levels of ammonia in the children's bloodstreams, they explained, "suggested that hepatic failure and resulting ammonia intoxication might be contributing factors in the pathogenesis of the encephalopathy." That is, the brain swelling (and its associated symptoms) might be the result of liver failure. That conclusion had significant consequences for the development of methods to diagnose Reye's syndrome, to treat it, and to determine its cause.

As a diagnostic tool, Huttenlocher and his team's finding that children with Reye's syndrome had significantly elevated levels of ammonia offered a quick and easy way to screen for RS in patients that presented with at least some of its associated symptoms. At the time, Reye's syndrome was confirmed either at autopsy—by which time it was obviously too late for the diagnosis to be of any medical value—or with a liver biopsy, which was often difficult or impossible with a child that was vomiting violently or having convulsions. The focus on liver function made it possible, as Huttenlocher explained, "to separate cases of Reye's syndrome from most other severe, acute encephalopathies" because there appeared to be no ailment other than RS that presented with both brain swelling and elevated ammonia levels.

Huttenlocher and his colleagues recognized that the critical role that ammonia played in Reye's syndrome might also provide information to help identify its ultimate cause, a question that vexed physicians and researchers throughout the 1960s and 1970s and still elicits controversy today. They noted that a prodromal illness was documented in nearly all cases of Reye's syndrome in the literature. While the illness that preceded the development of the syndrome was most often influenza, there were also reported cases of echovirus type 2, Coxsackievirus type A, andeovirus type 3, chicken pox, and reovirus. If elevated levels of ammonia marked the transition between the prodromal illness and the development of Reye's syndrome, the origins of Reye's syndrome might be found in whatever led to the rise in ammonia. A role for ammonia would also clarify the relationship between the two key attributes of Reye's syndrome, encephalitis and fatty degeneration of the liver, because ammonia indicated liver dysfunction and its elevated levels would cause encephalitis. That is, Huttenlocher's discovery pointed to the liver as the starting point for the development of Reye's syndrome. Therefore, if ammonia were involved in causing encephalitis in patients with Reye's syndrome, successful treatments would have to combat the elevated levels of ammonia present in the patient's bloodstream.

Whatever therapies emerged, it was clear that early detection was key to their success. As Huttenlocher and his colleagues concluded in their 1969 article, "Early diagnosis is essential if any therapeutic attempts are to be made." The identification of elevated ammonia levels as both a diagnostic indicator of Reye's syndrome and a cause of the children's acute encephalitis was an important step in understanding and treating RS. The authors concluded by reporting that they had come to believe that the most appropriate therapy for children suffering from Reye's syndrome was a dramatic therapy called exchange transfusion.

In the 1960s, as pediatricians were just beginning to chronicle the hundreds, perhaps thousands, of children who contracted Reye's syndrome every year, another group of physicians had been dealing with an ailment that shared several important symptoms with RS but for which the cause was known. Hepatitis—inflammation of the liver caused by infection, exposure to toxins, and autoimmune disorders—sometimes failed to resolve itself and occasionally led to hepatic coma. The liver is capable of regenerating itself, so treatments for liver disorders often involve methods that allow the liver the time it needs to recuperate. Beginning in the late 1950s, physicians at several different hospitals around the world had experimented with exchange transfusions, hoping that the procedure would "remove sufficient 'toxic' substances to allow the patient to be kept alive for regeneration and recovery to take place." An exchange transfusion is a medical treatment whereby a patient's blood is slowly removed and replaced with donor blood or plasma that has been prewarmed to body temperature.

The first physicians to attempt to use exchange transfusions as therapy for hepatic coma were a group of South Africans, who reported in 1958 that they had been successful in a patient. In 1966, the same group published a paper in the *New England Journal of Medicine* reporting on seven patients who had fallen into hepatic comas and were treated with exchange transfusions. All seven had awoken from their comas, and five of them had recovered completely. (The other two had died from causes that were not directly associated with their hepatitis or the treatment.) That same year, a team of physicians in Boston reported on a single case of acute hepatic coma that had been successfully treated with a pair of exchange transfusions. In 1967, physicians in Seattle reported on five cases of liver disease in which they had used the procedure, but only one of the patients had survived; they still, however, considered exchange transfusions a potentially valuable therapeutic tool because all five cases were so dire that they had expected the patients to die.

Citing the research on the use of exchange transfusions in patients with liver failure, Huttenlocher and his colleagues decided to try replacing the blood of a child with Reye's syndrome with blood from a healthy donor. They had first considered using the technique on a patient with RS after reading a 1924 paper by A. P. Hart, a physician in Toronto, who had used the therapy on a newborn baby boy who had been born healthy and strong at birth, but quickly developed a severe case of jaundice. Six other baby boys of these parents had developed the same serious jaundice shortly after birth, and all six infants had died. Hart reported that "it seemed as though the condition must be due to some toxin circulating in the blood which was destroying the liver cells, and as both the parents and I felt that if something drastic was not done at once the child was certainly going to die as the six other previous male babies had done." Hart's patient survived and thrived, and exchange transfusions became a valuable tool in treating sickle-cell anemia, jaundice, and other liver disorders, especially in infants. Inspired by Hart's account, Huttenlocher and his colleagues stated that, given the high mortality rate of Reye's syndrome and the nature of the ailment, they had hoped the same procedure would prove useful in helping children with RS overcome their symptoms.

Of the ten children with Reye's syndrome described in Huttenlocher's 1969 paper, three were treated with exchange transfusions, enemas, and neomycin, an antibiotic that kills intestinal bacteria and helps maintain low ammonia levels. The results were not encouraging: two of the three patients died. However, like the deaths seen by the Seattle physicians, Huttenlocher and his colleagues reported that the two children in their study who died had exhibited signs of brain death prior to the start of treatment. They concluded, "Further therapeutic trials will have to be made before this form of treatment should be discarded as ineffective."

Three years later, in 1972, Huttenlocher published an article that described eight additional cases of Reye's syndrome that were treated with the protocol he had developed. Seven of the eight children had survived, which was a much higher survival rate than most other physicians at the time were seeing in Reye's syndrome patients. He believed that there were two reasons for the relatively high survival rate in his patients with RS: early detection and the exchange transfusion treatment that he and his colleagues had developed. All of the children who arrived at the hospital with a history of viral infection followed by vomiting, stupor, or delirium were given liver function tests to look for elevated levels of ammonia or indications of liver dysfunction.

The protocol that Huttenlocher developed allowed for rapid diagnosis in children who were at risk of developing life-threatening encephalitis and treatment of the underlying cause of the encephalitis—which was liver dysfunction and an accumulation of toxins in the bloodstream—before it threatened the child's life. Any child found to have high blood-ammonia values was immediately given a 10 percent glucose solution intravenously, cleansing enemas, and neomycin both by mouth and as suppositories. If the blood-ammonia levels were high (defined as 300 micrograms per 100 milliliters), suitable blood donors were sought. If there were signs of falling into a coma—if the child had lost consciousness but still showed response to pain—doctors initiated an exchange transfusion. In four of the eight new cases that Huttenlocher described, the children had received exchange transfusions, and all four of them survived despite the fact that three of them had fallen into comas. Exchange transfusions seemed to work, and their success pointed the way for the development of a protocol for treating children with Reye's syndrome and provided further evidence that Reye's syndrome began with impairments of the children's livers eventually leading to ammonia intoxication, encephalitis, and too often death.

Treating the Symptoms

The 1976 film on Reye's syndrome produced by Chicago's WBBN had featured two doctors, William Schubert and John Partin, who played an important role in both treating patients with RS and in helping develop and assess treatments. Both were physicians at the Cincinnati Children's Hospital, and they authored at least eighteen publications on Reye's syndrome throughout the 1970s and 1980s. Schubert was a pediatrician whose work focused on pediatric gastroenterology, the branch of medicine that focuses on the digestive system, and he was renowned for his work building the city's research and clinical institutions. He died in 2012, and it is clear from the tributes written about him that he was a tremendously effective physician, researcher, mentor, and institution builder. In retrospect, we can see that many of these qualities were entwined in his contributions to the treatment and study of Reye's syndrome.

Schubert appeared in the introduction of WBBN's film on Reye's syndrome, and the focus of the film was the effort that he and his colleagues made to treat patients with RS. Schubert told viewers that Reye's syndrome was "a mysterious illness" and that initial reports of it were received "with considerable skepticism by people in medicine." Schubert's and Partin's patients were then shown in various stages of illness, and funding for research on RS was a significant theme throughout the film. Partin said, "This is a fairly costly business because the machinery is expensive and also we need research workers and technicians. It is very expensive, and we are handicapped because we don't have enough money to be able to pursue even the ideas that have been generated here in the Children's Hospital Research Foundation." Five years earlier, the announcer explained, the National Institutes of Health had been unwilling to pay for research on Reye's syndrome because it said the illness was "not serious." By 1975, though, it funded RS research with about $400,000. Partin compared the investments in research on Reye's syndrome to the investigation of polio. "If we can find a cure," he said, "we would save money. Polio vaccine development, diphtheria vaccine development and similar things have really been profitable in the long run not only in terms of child health and salvage of children but also in real money." Behind an image of a screaming child surrounded by medical personnel, the announcer concluded, "So, until more money is spent, the suffering will continue and children here and elsewhere will continue to die, painfully and helplessly."

Schubert, Partin, and their colleagues at Cincinnati Children's Hospital did much to advance our knowledge of Reye's syndrome, and by the mid-1970s they had helped develop effective treatments for it. Their early work examined the structure of cells in the livers and brains of children with RS through the use of electron microscopes, which in the film Partin had specifically stated were expensive. In the 1980s, as the aspirin hypothesis grew to dominate public and professional discussions about Reye's syndrome, Schubert and Partin turned the focus of these studies to look at the effects of salicylates on the liver using the same methods and microscopes. Using Lovejoy's framework for the clinical staging of RS, the clinicians developed appropriate treatments for each stage of the illness. In the 1974 season—the one depicted in the film produced by WBBN—Cincinnati Children's Hospital treated twenty-six children with Reye's syndrome with tremendous success. Every one of the children survived that year's season of Reye's syndrome, although at least one had severe brain damage.

In 1975, Schubert and three colleagues published an extensive review of the state of knowledge of Reye's syndrome for *Disease-a-Month*, a monthly publication for primary care physicians. The thirty-page booklet described the ailment's clinical presentation, pathology, the biochemical changes found in patients, and possible causes and treatment. They recommended supportive therapy for all children suspected of having Reye's syndrome consisting of an IV for hydration and careful monitoring of the children's conditions. Earlier efforts to stabilize patients' blood-sugar levels with insulin had proven ineffective, they said, and "should be discarded." In its place they recommended Huttenlocher's exchange transfusions.

The physicians at Cincinnati Children's Hospital had first tried using exchange transfusions to treat Reye's syndrome in 1969, the same year that Huttenlocher had started using them. Over the previous six years they had treated nine patients with Reye's syndrome, using "general supportive measures, including 10–15% glucose infusion" through IVs, "but all nine had died." Facing such terrible odds, when a child presented in 1969, they decided to treat him with an exchange transfusion and found success. "Since 1969," they explained, "the procedure has been uniform once the decision is made to exchange." Children diagnosed with RS—usually with needle biopsies of their livers—have one or two large catheters placed into the right atriums of their hearts or the vena cava, the large veins that bring blood directly into the heart. Physicians completely exchanged each child's blood twice after the catheters were placed, then once a day after that.

Even more dramatic than blood exchanges were Schubert and his colleagues' technique for monitoring brain swelling. They would drill a hole into the patient's skull and place a catheter into the subdural space so they could chart their patients' intracranial pressures. From the early 1970s onward, clinicians and researchers recognized that "the status of intracranial pressure in Reye syndrome represents a major issue of fundamental importance in diagnosing the disease and treating the victims." With a close eye on the patient's intracranial pressure, physicians could then adopt already established techniques for controlling the pressures that rose as their patients' brains swelled. Drugs like dexamethasone reduced the water and sodium content in patient's brains. Mannitol, a sugar alcohol that is produced by hydrogenating fructose, and urea were valuable tools in reducing intracranial pressure. In the 1980s, physicians experimented with several drugs—including thiopenone, legalon, and lokhein—to treat cerebral edema in patients suffering from Reye's syndrome.

When drugs alone could not control rising intracranial pressures in children suffering from Reye's syndrome, some physicians adopted more aggressive tactics. For example, in 1982 a group of physicians from the Children's Hospital of Philadelphia described sixty-seven children they had treated for Reye's syndrome between 1977 and 1981. Forty-five of the patients' illnesses progressed to a point that the team defined as "severe Reye's syndrome," identified by the patient having lost consciousness and having developed an abnormal, stiff posture with bent arms, clenched fists and legs held straight out (called decorticate posture or "mummy baby"). In 1977 and 1978 they had treated twenty patients with Reye's syndrome that had progressed to the severe stages with combinations of drug-induced comas, hypothermia, transfusions, and the administration of drugs to reduce intracranial pressure. Beginning in 1979, they treated another twenty-three patients with both drug-induced comas and by inducing hypothermia. They had hypothesized that by artificially inducing coma with phenobarbital and by reducing their patients' temperatures, they could protect the children's brains from the side effects of swelling. Unfortunately, despite the relatively dramatic interventions, the outcomes were not significantly better. They concluded, "We failed to demonstrate a significant difference in outcome with early institution of pentobarbital/hypothermia therapy compared to therapy used only in response to rises in [intracranial pressure]." Given the high mortality rate of children whose Reye's syndrome progressed to the later stages, some physicians—with consent from desperate parents—continued to use drug-induced comas as therapy for RS. A 1981 *Los Angeles Times* story quoted the doctor of a fourteen-month-old girl who was fighting for her life; "What happens is the brain is put to sleep waiting for the toxic effects of Reye's to dissipate." Later authors, however, agreed that the approach was not recommended because it might "have a deleterious effect on the metabolic problems associated with this disease."

Perhaps the most dramatic effort to reduce intracranial pressure in children with Reye's syndrome was decompressive craniectomy, and a description from even a single case demonstrates just how desperate parents and physicians were as they watched a child's condition worsen. Sometimes called trepanning, decompressive craniectomy is the removal of a section of the skull in order to prevent the brain from crushing itself as intracranial pressures increase. First performed on children with RS in the late 1960s, it tended to be a treatment of last resort and was used in children whose symptoms had advanced to stage V. Schubert and his colleagues described their experience with the treatment at the end of their 1976 review of the state of knowledge of Reye's syndrome. The procedure had, they said, "been lifesaving in one of our patients." In 1974, a six-year-old girl presented at the hospital with classic symptoms of Reye's syndrome. She had been well before contracting an upper respiratory infection that included a runny nose and a cough. As she began to overcome the routine childhood illness, she started vomiting violently, grew irritable, and developed a "staggering gait and staring gaze." She was admitted to the hospital and meningoencephalitis was diagnosed, but a lumbar puncture failed to confirm the diagnosis. Within hours she fell into a deep coma and was unresponsive to pain. Her heart rate was fast, and her pupils were dilated and sluggish to respond to light. The laboratory results suggested (and the needle biopsy of her liver confirmed) that she suffered from Reye's syndrome. Schubert and his colleagues attempted the usual treatment of exchange transfusion, but the girl's condition worsened. "It was considered that the irreversible consequences of severe brain swelling were imminent and craniectomy was undertaken as a life-saving measure." Over the next two days sections from either side of the girl's skull were removed, while exchange transfusions continued every twelve hours. Her physicians later described how, "in spite of a stormy course due to pulmonary complications and a bleeding Cushing's ulcer which required surgical intervention, the child is recovering." Ten months after she fell ill, she "assists nurses in caring for infants on the surgical ward where she likes to play doctor." But she did not survive Reye's syndrome unscathed. About a year after she was admitted to the hospital, the once healthy and normal six-year-old tested with an IQ of 80 and had "demonstrated perceptual-motor difficulties."

Given their obvious personal and professional investments in children with Reye's syndrome, physicians like Schubert and Partin were painfully frustrated by the suffering, damage, and deaths they saw in these children, especially as the number of cases accumulated year after year. These frustrations were evident when the authors concluded the case description of their six-year-old patient by recounting the girl's exasperation with her now-limited abilities: "She could copy a circle, cross and square but she failed to copy a triangle and she refused to attempt the divided rectangle, throwing the crayon across the room instead."

From Therapy to Prevention

By the late 1970s, clinicians had developed both the diagnostic tools and the therapies they needed to treat patients that presented with the symptoms of Reye's syndrome. By then, parents, pediatricians, and family doctors were relatively well informed about the warning signs of Reye's syndrome, especially in the Great Lakes states where the ailment was most frequently diagnosed. Physicians and parents had developed a relatively high index of suspicion for the disorder because of widespread media coverage of the occasional cases of RS that had appeared and because of the increasing visibility of local chapters of the National Reye's Syndrome Foundation (NRSF).

Founded in Bryan, Ohio, in 1974, the NRSF was an organized movement of citizens—most of them parents of children affected by Reye's syndrome—that sought to eradicate the ailment through public awareness of its symptoms, identification of possible causes, and the development of effective treatments. John and Terri Freudenberger and Michael and Susan Huffman created it after their children had contracted RS in the early 1970s. The Freudenbergers' daughter, Tiffini, had died early on a Sunday morning in 1973 from the symptoms of Reye's syndrome. A year later, the Huffmans' daughter, Stephanie, developed RS and survived. Later that year the parents formed the foundation "to raise funds for Reye's syndrome research and treatment, and to provide funding toward the cure and prevention of this mysterious disease." The local chapter of the Jaycees were early supporters of the organization, contributing manpower and financial donations to publish educational brochures for distribution in schools.

Throughout the 1970s and 1980s, the NRSF published a scientific journal, hosted medical and scientific conferences, and encouraged the emergence of local chapters. Annual holiday card sales, the cooperation of the American Legion, and increasingly large donations from corporate sponsors and individuals allowed the foundation to provide over twenty grants to researchers and to continue its efforts to inform parents and health-care providers about warning signs of Reye's syndrome. Dudley Moore, Dick Van Dyke, and Bill Cosby were all public supporters of the NRSF, and the foundation was increasingly active in encouraging federal and state legislatures to promote awareness of the illness. At its peak, NRSF had nearly eighty local chapters around the country, all of which eventually merged with the national organization as the illness disappeared throughout the late 1980s and early 1990s. Today, the NRSF still operates from its headquarters in Bryan, spreading awareness of the warning signs of Reye's syndrome and encouraging parents to avoid giving their children aspirin, which it states is a possible cause of the deadly illness.

The 1980 season for Reye's syndrome, which lasted through the first four months of the year, witnessed 555 reported cases in the United States alone, the highest ever reported annual number before and since. Mortality rates had fallen to under 20 percent, still frighteningly high, and almost every possible cause that had been suggested had been disputed or outright rejected by most authorities. Now our story shifts out of the hospital and on to the work of the CDC's Epidemic Intelligence Service, the same organization that had employed George Johnson when he had identified sixteen cases of what he called an "encephalitis-like disease" in 1963. And 1980 was the year aspirin became the focus of many people's concerns about Reye's syndrome.

CHAPTER FIVE

The Aspirin Hypothesis

THROUGHOUT THE 1960S AND 1970S, as physicians and scientists struggled to find the cause of Reye's syndrome, they had occasionally pointed fingers at over-the-counter drugs like acetaminophen (better known by its trade name, Tylenol) and aspirin. Liver dysfunction seemed to be at the root of Reye's syndrome and the majority of the cases had no virus or toxin in common; over-the-counter drugs were one of the few common denominators among most of the children who had contracted RS. In the United States at that time, aspirin was by far the most widely used drug to lower children's fevers and to treat their minor aches and pains. It was given to so many children that researchers were hard pressed to find children who had the kind of prodromal illnesses that sometimes developed into Reye's syndrome but had not been given aspirin. In addition, aspirin had a long safety record, and from the start it simply made no sense to think it might cause such a deadly illness.

Aspirin's history stretches back to antiquity, and in modern times it had been widely and safely used for nearly a century before Reye's syndrome emerged. Aspirin is the common name for acetylsalicylic acid, and salicylic acid is the main metabolite in aspirin. So in discussions about a possible relationship between aspirin and Reye's syndrome, the terms "aspirin," "salicylic acid," and "acetylsalicylic acid" were used interchangeably. Plant extracts from spiraea and willow bark contain salicylic acid and for thousands of years have been known to help relieve pain and reduce fevers. Archaeologists have found 4,000-year-old Assyrian clay tablets that describe the use of willow leaves to relieve pain and inflammation. The Babylonian Code of Hammurabi (c. 1750 B.C.) included similar information, and the ancient Egyptians used willow leaves to treat inflammation. In the fifth century B.C., Hippocrates recommended chewing willow bark to relieve fever and pain and a brew of willow leaves to ease the pains of childbirth, and five hundred years later the Greek physician Dioscorides repeated Hippocrates's recommendations. Pliny and Galen both treated wounds and ulcers with willow leaves. But it was not until 1971—when aspirin was shown to interfere with the synthesis of fatty acids that cause inflammation—that the exact pharmacology of the substance from the willow tree was finally known.

From the 1850s through the 1890s, European chemists worked to isolate and describe salicylic acid, which was widely recognized as effective in cooling fevers and reducing pain. However, salicylic acid irritates the stomach and frequently causes nausea and a ringing in the ears. In the late 1890s, chemists in Germany working at Bayer AG began experimenting with acetylsalicylic acid, which is produced by reacting salicylic acid with methanol. The resulting product lowered fevers and reduced pain, but did not seem to have the adverse affects on patients' stomachs and ears that salicylic acid produced.

For decades, credit for development of the new drug has been given to Felix Hoffman, but Arthur Eichengrün later claimed that he was the lead investigator and that his role in the development of aspirin had been expunged by the Nazi regime during the 1930s. Eichengrün, a Bayer chemist in the 1890s, left the company in 1908 to establish his own factory in Berlin, finding tremendous success producing flame-resistant materials with acetyl cellulose and pioneering the process of injection molding plastics. Despite having amassed considerable wealth, Eichengrün's fortunes declined precipitously in the 1930s, as the Nazi party excluded Jews like him from many aspects of German society, politics, and business. A 1934 history of chemical engineering credited Hoffman with the discovery of acetylsalicylic acid, and Eichengrün was unable to assert his role in the new drug for fear of Nazi retaliation. He was eventually interned in the concentration camp at Theresienstadt for fourteen months before being liberated by the Soviets in 1945. Shortly before he died in 1949, Eichengrün published an account of his invention of aspirin, which was largely ignored for the next fifty years. It was not until

2000, when the historian Walter Sneader published an article in the *British Medical Journal* exploring the history of aspirin, that Eichengrün was rightly credited.

Bayer had quickly recognized the commercial value of acetylsalicylic acid and by 1899 was selling Aspirin under trademark around the world. Its popularity quickly grew, and it proved to be a tremendously effective and profitable drug. As part of the reparations for World War I, Bayer lost the trademark for Aspirin in France, Russia, the United Kingdom, and the United States, and aspirin has since been the generic name for acetylsalicylic acid. It has long been marketed as a "wonder drug," and its usefulness as a pain reliever and fever reducer has lately been augmented by research showing that it reduces the risk of cardiovascular disease and recent findings that it helps prevent cancer. By the 1960s, aspirin's safety seemed assured. Americans alone bought about 9 million pounds of the little white pills every year, and the drug generated significant profits for aspirin manufacturers. Three generations had relied on aspirin, and it seemed to have relatively few side effects when used for occasional relief of pain or fever. It should have come as no surprise, therefore, that physicians and parents might have been skeptical about alleged links between aspirin and Reye's syndrome even as they ardently sought the cause of Reye's syndrome. As we will see, many physicians doubted the association and resented government efforts in the 1980s to warn parents against giving aspirin to children with viral illnesses. But parents—especially those living in regions that saw higher numbers of cases of Reye's syndrome—quickly adopted the aspirin hypothesis as a suitable explanation of *the* cause of Reye's syndrome, even though no scientific research demonstrated a causal relationship between the two.

Early Accusations

While is was hard for most people to imagine that aspirin might be the cause of the apparently new syndrome described by Reye and his colleagues, from the very start aspirin had been mentioned as a suspect by some researchers. In 1962, a year before the publications of Reye's and Johnson's articles, Edward A. Mortimer, Jr., and Martha Lipson Lepow described four infants who had died shortly after being admitted to the hospital. They all had significant swelling of the brain and fatty degeneration of the liver, precisely the same symptoms that would become the hallmark of Reye's syndrome only a few years later. Aside from living in the same region of the country and contracting varicella, Mortimer and Lepow found no similarities among the children that would have explained the sudden onset of such similar symptoms and their eventual deaths, except "the administration of large amounts of salicylates to the infants for a period of several days preceding the appearance of hypoglycemia." They hypothesized that the children's low blood-sugar levels were the result of a combination of varicella infection, salicylates, and their inability to keep down food. "It seemed possible," they wrote, "that the carbohydrate reserves of these infants might have been depleted by 3 factors: the stress of the varicella, decreased intake because of fasting and vomiting, and the administration of salicylates over several days." Mortimer and Lepow pursued their hypothesis with an experiment on rats to see if aspirin could affect the liver in such a way that the rats were unable to maintain adequately high blood-sugar levels. They administered sodium salicylate to fasting rats, tested their blood-sugar levels, then administered epinephrine and retested their blood-sugar levels. If aspirin was partially responsible for the deaths of these four infants, they believed they would find that the blood sugars would be lower in the rats that had received sodium salicylate than they were in the controls. They found that the rats that had received large doses of aspirin "exhibited significantly lower blood sugar levels and diminished responses to epinephrine than fasted control rats." As a result, they "concluded that the hypoglycemia observed in the four infants may possibly have been related to salicylates."

Most of the early authors who had raised the possibility that salicylates might be the cause of the symptoms that came to be associated with Reye's syndrome focused on the possibility that the children had overdosed on aspirin. For example, the three physicians from the Transvaal Memorial Hospital for Children in Johannesburg, South Africa, who had suggested the name "white liver" disease for what would eventually be called Reye's syndrome reported, "Where salicylate was considered as a possible cause of the disease, the serum-salicylate level was never raised to more than mild-to-moderate levels." Their framing of the issue by the amount of aspirin the children had consumed—rather than by the fact that they had consumed any aspirin at all—demonstrated their assumption that normal levels of aspirin were not harmful and thus would have played no role in the children's illnesses.

The first to suggest that normal doses of aspirin might, in some children, induce the symptoms of Reye's syndrome was a physician in Birmingham, England, H. McC. Giles. He knew of nine local cases that conformed to Reye's description, and he wrote to the *Lancet* "to suggest that salicylates may be involved." Giles had identified a total of thirty-one cases of Reye's syndrome locally and in the medical literature, and he found that at least fifteen of them had received aspirin and another six may have received it. The actual percentage of children given aspirin might, Giles said, be much higher than authorities presumed. He had learned that three of the four cases he had treated had received aspirin only after "close and direct questioning elicited the fact that it had been given." Giles posited that it might be that "in some children the enzyme system involved in carbohydrate metabolism is hypersensitive." He concluded, "It seems worth urging that investigation of Reye's syndrome should include a very careful and determined inquiry concerning aspirin or salicylate administration."

Given that ultimately aspirin would be implicated as a cause of Reye's syndrome, my interest was piqued when I read case accounts from the first half of the twentieth century of children dying from acute encephalopathy who had received aspirin in the course of their illnesses. For example, in the sixteen case reports of "acute encephalopathies of obscure origin" that the researchers from Massachusetts General Hospital published in 1961, two of the ill children reportedly received aspirin in the course of their prodromal illness. More telling, however, was the fact that the authors explained that the most effective (and presumably widely used) method of controlling the children's seizures was to administer aspirin to lower their fevers. That fact alone suggests that far more than two of the sixteen ill children had actually received aspirin.

In 1965, four physicians at the University of Washington in Seattle published a detailed case study that demonstrated the potential for aspirin to cause lethargy, irritability, and seizures—all symptoms associated with Reye's syndrome. They reported on a twenty-two-month-old boy who had struggled most of his young life with a variety of health problems, including very low blood sugars. He had suffered three seizures, one each at sixteen, eighteen, and twenty months of age. Beginning when he was about five months old, his mother had administered one or two baby aspirin (about 60 to 150 milligrams) each day as a treatment for "irritability, teething, sleeplessness, etc." The physicians admitted the child to the hospital so they could perform two aspirin-response tests that could help determine whether the aspirin therapy and the child's very low blood sugars were related. After fasting the child for eight hours, they administered 300 milligrams (about the equivalent of four baby aspirin). The tests had to be stopped because the boy's blood sugar dropped precipitously and on one of the two tests he suffered another seizure. Because of the results of the aborted tests, the doctors suspended the child's daily dose of aspirin; his symptoms subsided. They also included in their report short descriptions of two other cases—one fatal—they had seen in the previous eighteen months of young children in which aspirin and severely depressed blood sugars seemed to coincide. They concluded, "On the basis of the experience with these three patients in a relatively brief period of time, it would seem that perhaps the occurrence of hypoglycemia following salicylate ingestion is more common than the paucity of reports in the literature would imply." Never, though, did they connect their findings with Reye's "clinicopathological entity of unknown ætiology."

Given the results of the experiments with rats that were performed by Mortimer and Lepow as well as the experience of the young patient studied by the physicians at the University of Washington, it seemed plausible that at least some young children suffered from severely depressed blood sugars when they were given aspirin. This could account for at least some of the symptoms associated with Reye's syndrome, especially when the low blood sugar appeared with fasting, diarrhea, or vomiting. It had been known since the late nineteenth century that aspirin could significantly affect carbohydrate metabolism. Before the introduction of insulin therapy, very large—and sometimes toxic—doses of salicylates had been administered to some diabetic patients to help reduce their blood sugars. Experiments on rats in the 1940s and 1950s provided additional evidence that salicylates and aspirin both appeared to have an effect on the animals' ability to metabolize carbohydrates.

By the mid-1960s, Reye's syndrome had become widely enough known among physicians to prompt them to publish reports of cases that appeared similar to what Reye and Johnson had first reported in 1963. Some early reports pointed to the possibility that aspirin was involved in some way. For example, in a 1968 report of twenty-one cases that appeared at the children's hospital in Toronto, Ontario over a twelve-year period, the hospital's chief resident stated that physicians there suspected that the afflicted children had been overdosed with aspirin because they had been hyperventilating, a common symptom of salicylate intoxication. Many of the children had been administered aspirin to control their fevers before admission to the hospital, and ten of the twenty-one sick children had the salicylate levels in their blood measured. All ten tested within the normal range for therapeutic doses of aspirin and far below the levels expected for someone who has overdosed on aspirin. In hindsight, because we know that the aspirin hypothesis would come to play such a significant role in later discussions about the onset of Reye's syndrome, this 1968 article seems prescient. But it discussed the possible role of salicylates only very briefly, and the author concluded that the measured levels were relatively low, so he concluded that it was unlikely that the cause of the children's fatty livers was iatrogenic—that is, caused by a medical intervention, in this case aspirin—because no common single drug was administered to every child.

An authoritative rejection of any notion of a link between aspirin and Reye's syndrome emerged in 1970 with the publication in *Pediatrics* of the results of a selective epidemiologic study of Reye's syndrome in sixty-two cases over a thirty-month period. Physicians from the viral diseases branch of the U.S. Public Health Service summarized their findings from a study of cases from the mainland United States and Puerto Rico in the late 1960s. Included in their study was an analysis of the possible role of salicylates in the patients' illnesses. They found that slightly more than half of the children were known to have ingested aspirin. They ultimately stated, "Considerable negative epidemiologic evidence in the present series of cases indicates that most, if not all, cases of Reye's syndrome in the United States are etiologically unrelated to exogenous toxins or common medications." Aspirin, the U.S. Public Health Service therefore concluded in 1970, was not the cause of Reye's syndrome.

But other government agencies did not agree, and the first official pronouncement that there might be a link between aspirin and Reye's syndrome came six years later, when the U.S. Food and Drug Administration published a report in the *FDA Drug Bulletin* recommending broadly against the use of all antiemetics—drugs used to reduce nausea and vomiting—as well as aspirin, acetaminophen, and antibiotics in children suspected of having Reye's syndrome. There was no evidence in the literature the report cited that demonstrated a link between any of these common medications and Reye's syndrome. Rather, the FDA—which was charged with ensuring the safety of drugs—suggested that antiemetics, aspirin, acetaminophen, or antibiotics might be involved in the origins of Reye's syndrome because almost every other possible cause had been ruled out. Given the history of prodromal illnesses in the vast majority of cases, a considerable number of different over-the-counter drugs were given to children just before they began exhibiting signs of RS. This was hardly a valid reason to implicate aspirin, though. More evidence was obviously necessary before any conclusions could be reached about the possible relationship of over-the-counter drugs and Reye's syndrome. Late in 1980, just such evidence began to emerge from the work of the Epidemic Intelligence Service, a small army of public health researchers that had been sent into the field by the CDC.

The Epidemic Intelligence Service

Researchers and physicians working as officers for the Epidemic Intelligence Service had long been searching for the source of Reye's syndrome. George Johnson, the EIS officer in North Carolina in the early 1960s, had identified and published a description of the illness nearly simultaneously with Reye and his colleagues and then reported on it at the annual EIS meeting. Throughout the 1960s and 1970s, EIS officers at the CDC's headquarters in Atlanta and those working with state public health officials had provided surveillance of new cases of Reye's syndrome as they developed methods for helping identify its cause. Thomas Glick, an EIS officer in the late 1960s, had set up the first informal surveillance network for Reye's syndrome in 1967 and had identified sixty-two cases of it in the mainland United States and Puerto Rico over a three-year period. He had also been the lead author on the 1970 report from the U.S. Public Health Service that had rejected suggestions of a relationship between RS and aspirin. But his efforts to identify the source of the illness laid the groundwork for later research on the subject that generated opposite conclusions.

In the latter half of the 1970s, as the officials at the FDA started suggesting that there might be a connection between commonly used medicines and Reye's syndrome, EIS officers apparently began to gradually shift their thinking on the issue. Lawrence Corey, an EIS officer in the mid-1970s, published a number of papers on diagnostic criteria for RS, comparisons of different therapeutic interventions, and the frequency of particular illnesses prodromal to Reye's syndrome. He was lead author on a 1977 article in *Pediatrics* that, among other things, briefly explored the possibility of a link between aspirin and RS. In their analysis of the 379 cases of Reye's syndrome reported in 1974, the authors had found that patients who had consumed salicylates during their prodromal illness fared no better or worse than those who had not. They also recognized that some previous studies had found that all of the cases they studied had received salicylates before the onset of the symptoms of RS. While they could not determine from their data if there was a correlation between aspirin and Reye's syndrome, they did assert that "only an analysis of aspirin use in children who develop uncomplicated influenza B infection vs. those who develop influenza B–associated Reye's syndrome will further elucidate the role salicylates may have in the pathogenesis of this syndrome." Given the ubiquity of aspirin, it would have been difficult to find a sufficient number of children who not received aspirin during a minor illness in order to create such a study. However, as parents began using acetaminophen in place of aspirin in the late 1970s, the possibility emerged for a comparative study of the children who did and did not receive aspirin during the course of a normal childhood illness.

The first strong epidemiological evidence implicating aspirin emerged from a small study conducted by Karen Starko, an EIS officer in Phoenix, Arizona. During an outbreak of influenza A in December 1978, Starko identified seven children who had been hospitalized with Reye's syndrome. Two of them—an eleven-year-old and a twelve-year-old—had died. Within four weeks after the children had been hospitalized, Starko interviewed their parents as well as the parents of sixteen other children who had also been ill but had not developed symptoms of Reye's syndrome. She asked detailed questions about the medications that were given and their amounts. Starko later explained the children "were perfectly healthy before they got the flu," so she had thought it "logical to hypothesize that whatever was causing RS happened between the onset of flu and the severe vomiting." That was a "defined and narrow period of four days," allowing her to create a case-control study that focused on "symptoms of the virus, medications, and a few other exposures like pets, vaccinations, [and] home heating." Salicylate-containing drugs were the only statistically significant factor that emerged when she compared the children who had contracted RS with the case controls that she had chosen from among the children's classmates.

In the spring of 1979, Starko discussed her findings with Lawrence Schonberger, a supervisor at the CDC who ran a surveillance system for RS and coordinated the EIS officers' work on Reye's syndrome. Starko's work provided the first substantial clue that there might be a relationship between aspirin and RS, and Schonberger was sufficiently intrigued to share her initial findings with other EIS officers who were studying Reye's syndrome. After speaking to Eugene Hurwitz, who was leading a large study on Reye's syndrome in Ohio, Schonberger asked Hurwitz to change the Ohio study to focus on the treatment of the antecedent illness and to play particular attention to aspirin.

Starko had not been specifically looking for evidence of a relationship between aspirin and Reye's syndrome, and when she began interviewing the parents of children afflicted with RS, she had known relatively little about the ailment. So when the ingestion of aspirin emerged as the only statically significant difference between the children who had developed Reye's syndrome and the children who had not, she turned to the published medical reports to see if she could find supporting evidence of a relationship between RS and aspirin. Just as nearly two decades earlier George Johnson had spent "three long and lonesome days during the middle of the investigation in the University of North Carolina medical library," Starko settled into the Maricopa County Medical Society Library to search the literature for clues that aspirin might have some relationship with Reye's syndrome. At the urging of her supervisor at the CDC, Lyle Conrad, in September 1979 she wrote to the Armed Forces Institute of Pathology in Washington to ask if they had encountered any cases of salicylate poisoning that produced symptoms similar to Reye's syndrome. Two weeks later she received from the institute details of eleven cases of acute salicylic poisoning in infants and children, all of which presented with the small fat droplets within the liver cells that were characteristic of Reye's syndrome. "I wanted to scream," she remembered thinking, "This was it!"

Starko found it was much easier to convince Schonberger of the possibility of a relationship between aspirin and Reye's syndrome than to convince the editors of medical journals. In September 1979, on the heels of hearing from the Armed Forces Institute of Pathology, she applied to present a paper on her initial findings at the American Public Health Association's annual meeting. It was rejected. A few months later, she submitted a paper to the *Lancet*, which also rejected it. Finally, late in the spring of 1980, she found some success in publicizing her findings. In April she presented at the meeting of Epidemic Intelligence Service officers, and two months later a report appeared in the CDC's *Morbidity and Mortality Weekly Report* on the association between aspirin and Reye's syndrome. Written in large part by Lawrence Schonberger, it was the first in what he would later describe as "gradually stronger warnings against the use of salicylates to treat children with an influenza-like or varicella illness." Later that spring, *Pediatrics* agreed to publish Starko's findings, which appeared in the December 1980 issue of the journal.

In the paper in *Pediatrics*, Starko and her colleagues described how they had found that children who had contracted Reye's syndrome "took more medications during their prodrome than did control children throughout their illness." In total, the children who contracted Reye's syndrome took about twice as much medicine as did the control subjects, and the additional drugs consisted almost entirely of salicylate-containing medications. The children that developed RS and the controls took on average about 1.5 medications, but the children that developed Reye's syndrome each took on average an additional 1.7 medications that contained salicylates. In total, the controls took about one-third as much salicylate-containing medicine as did the children who developed Reye's syndrome.

Starko and her colleagues recognized that, despite the strength of their findings, their study had a number of weaknesses. It had enrolled only a small number of children, and the nature of the children's illnesses caused a great deal of stress on the parents, which could easily have affected their ability to recall accurately the types and amounts of medications they had given to their children. The researchers had not definitively ascertained the children's prodromal illnesses, and they could not say for certain that the children who had developed Reye's syndrome and the children in the control group actually had suffered from the same illnesses. Nonetheless, they asserted, "our data indicate that salicylate should be further evaluated as a possible cause of Reye's syndrome." The authors concluded, "Until studies further evaluating this relationship are completed, we suggest that caution be exercised in giving salicylate to children with an otherwise benign illness."

It took the better part of a year for reactions to Starko and her colleagues' paper to appear in print. By the fall of 1981, a slew of letters to the editor appeared in *Pediatrics*, and almost every one of them rejected the authors' conclusion that there might be a relationship between aspirin and Reye's syndrome. The first came from William M. Young, a pediatrician in Fayetteville, Tennessee, who complained that the only thing the team had proved was "that the sicker the child is the more salicylates his parents give him." Obviously fearing the loss of a valuable weapon in the pediatrician's arsenal, Young asked, "In this era of therapeutic nihilism, are we not to be left with aspirin?" In the same issue, two pediatricians from the Indiana University School of Medicine wrote to say that they had reviewed the case files from sixty-eight cases of Reye's syndrome that had appeared at their hospital since 1973 and reported that salicylate levels had been tested in the majority of cases. The results, they said, were "hardly noteworthy," so they were dismissive of the aspirin hypothesis and pointed to significant visual differences in the livers of children with aspirin-induced liver damage as compared to the liver damage seen in children with Reye's syndrome. Like Young, they worried that increasing public awareness of the aspirin hypothesis would lead to increased use of acetaminophen to treat fevers. They concluded, "We consider acetaminophen potentially more hepatotoxic than aspirin." Two Canadian pediatricians wrote with similar findings from the twenty-seven cases of Reye's syndrome they had encountered in Toronto between 1973 and 1978. "The findings in these patients," they wrote, "do not support a role of salicylates as a causative agent in Reye's syndrome."

Starko and C. George Ray, one of her coauthors on the original paper, responded directly to the two pediatricians from the Indiana University School of Medicine. They asserted that Reye's syndrome was something different from an aspirin overdose, and thus the level of salicylates in the bloodstreams of the patients with Reye's syndrome were likely well within the range of normal doses. This, they wrote, "does not eliminate the possibility that the disease is drug induced or drug enhanced." They relied on recent findings from studies in Ohio and Michigan that were released after their paper had been published to support their own findings and called for studies that could thoroughly explore "in a scientific manner" why it appeared that the children that contracted Reye's syndrome seemed to take aspirin more frequently and in greater amounts than did the children who did not develop RS. They concluded by addressing the "therapeutic dilemma" that their work might pose to pediatricians. Starko and Ray explained that, despite their widespread use in children with viral infections, there was no evidence that either aspirin or acetaminophen helped children recover more quickly from their illnesses. "In fact," they wrote, "overzealous therapy may be deleterious to the patient." Quoting Thomas Sydenham, a seventeenth-century English physician, they concluded, "Fever is Nature's engine which she brings into the field to remove her enemy." Drugs like aspirin might relieve some patients' discomfort, lower fevers, and ease parents' concerns, but they did not speed a child's recovery from a viral illness.

The same year that Starko and her team from the CDC published the results of their small study in Arizona, eight researchers from the Ohio State Department of Health published the results of their five-year retrospective study of the 190 Ohio residents diagnosed with Reye's syndrome between 1973 and 1977. Their goal was to add to the relatively small but growing body of literature on the relationship between RS and the viral illnesses that typically preceded it. Several researchers had already identified influenza B as the most common prodromal illness in cases of Reye's syndrome, and still others had identified cases that seemed to have started with influenza A, chicken pox, or a handful of other viral illnesses. The virus that preceded the onset of the more serious symptoms of RS was obviously significant, as it was relatively uncommon to find cases of Reye's syndrome that lacked a prodromal illness. The Ohio researchers hoped that their analysis would "provide population-based data about Reye syndrome, including data from periods of time when epidemic influenza B was absent from the community."

To acquire data for their study, the researchers had contacted every hospital in Ohio that either had more than five hundred beds or more than forty pediatric beds and asked them to provide the medical records of every patient with Reye's syndrome that had been diagnosed before January 1, 1978. They studied 190 cases that fit the criteria and found that 20.5 percent had had chicken pox before the onset of symptoms of RS, 62.6 percent had had some sort of upper respiratory virus, 16.8 percent had suffered from any one of a variety of other illnesses, and 1.6 percent (three patients) had had no clinical illness before contracting Reye's syndrome. The team focused on the 151 patients who had an upper respiratory or some other virus, but not chicken pox. They found that there was a strong temporal relationship between outbreaks of influenza B and Reye's syndrome—that is, when there were more cases of influenza B in an area, there were more cases of Reye's syndrome, too.

There was nothing in the original Ohio study about medications or any relationship of a drug or toxin to Reye's syndrome; however, two of the researchers on the team that had conducted the study—Thomas Halpin and Francis Holtzhauer—continued to work with the data the group had collected. They interviewed the families of patients and controls from the initial study, asking questions about the medications the children had received during and shortly before their illnesses. Their findings were startling, and as they prepared to publish the results of their work, they made a brief report to the CDC that was published in the *Morbidity and Mortality Weekly Report*. When they compared the children who had contracted Reye's syndrome with the control group, the team found a significant difference in the use of two medications, salicylates and acetaminophen. Of the children who had contracted Reye's syndrome, 97 percent of them had taken medicines that contained salicylates during their prodromal illnesses. Among the controls, only 71 percent had taken a salicylate-containing medication during their prodromal illness. The results for acetaminophen were the opposite; only 16 percent of the children that eventually developed Reye's syndrome had taken acetaminophen during their prodromal illness, compared to 32 percent of the controls.

The editors of the *Morbidity and Mortality Weekly Report* attached a long note to the relatively short descriptions of the initial findings in Arizona and Ohio as well as reports of initial findings from some work done in Michigan. The suggestion that medications taken during the antecedent illness could play a role in the origins of Reye's syndrome, they wrote, had long lingered in the medical literature. However, by far the greater part of the editors' note consisted of comments on the studies' shortcomings. They described a "number of potential problems" that "are encountered when conducting and analyzing such studies," including difficulties in obtaining comparable and accurate medication histories, the possibility that children had suffered from undiagnosed illnesses, and difficulty in identifying cases with similar antecedent illnesses. Nonetheless, the editors concluded by reminding readers of the FDA's 1976 warning against giving acetaminophen, salicylates, or antiemetics to children with vomiting and a viral illness and asserting that the evidence from Arizona, Ohio, and Michigan—even though it was imperfect—meant that "parents should be advised to use caution when administering salicylates to treat children with viral illnesses, particularly chickenpox and influenza-like illnesses." The studies in Arizona, Ohio, and Michigan were only preliminary. But they encouraged EIS officers to look more closely at aspirin now that they were able to find patients who suffered minor childhood illnesses and did not receive aspirin, children they could compare to children who developed the much more serious symptoms associated with RS. On the eve of the rapid disappearance of the ailment, EIS officers in Michigan conducted the most thorough study investigating the possible relationship between aspirin and Reye's syndrome.

The Michigan Study

Michigan experienced some of the highest numbers of reported cases ever of Reye's syndrome of any state, and residents had grown especially fearful of RS as reports of it regularly appeared in local newspapers. For example, a 1974 article in the Benton Harbor *News-Palladium* described the deaths from Reye's syndrome of several children in Michigan, including a six-year-old boy from Mendon, a seven-year-old boy from Sturgis, and a thirteen-year-old girl from Coldwater. On the same page was an Associated Press story that stated that during the previous year, "Michigan reported the most cases [of Reye's syndrome], 27, followed by Ohio with 15 and Wisconsin with 14." A CDC official explained that the reported number of cases was certainly much lower than the actual number "because the disease is not a reportable disease as far as the Public Health Service is concerned, but the CDC asked state public health departments to make reports because of the increase in cases of the disease last winter." The lack of a formal reporting system was a significant problem for the physicians and researchers who were trying to understand RS and its causes better.

Spurred by public concern, in 1978 Michigan was the first state to enact a law requiring the reporting of all cases of Reye's syndrome to local and state departments of health. The Critical Health Problems Reporting Act was signed into law in the summer of 1978 and required that cases of Reye's syndrome, lead poisoning, and any disease, condition or procedure "determined by the director to be of particular concern or importance as a critical health problem" be reported not more than ten days after diagnosis. The reporting system allowed health officials to have much better surveillance of Reye's syndrome and the public learned about even more cases of the mysterious ailment. Small-town newspapers in the state continued, year after year, to print devastating stories about healthy young children struck with RS. The result was increased pressure on public health officials in the state to find the source of the illness as quickly as possible.

Empowered by the state's new reporting act, Ronald Waldman, an EIS officer working in Michigan, led the effort there to identify the cause or causes of Reye's syndrome. Waldman was a Swiss-trained physician who went on to earn a master's degree in public health from Johns Hopkins University in 1979 and then joined the EIS program. During the 1980 season, eighty-three cases of Reye's syndrome were reported to the Michigan Department of Public Health. Waldman and his colleagues interviewed the parents of twenty-five of the children as well as the parents of forty-six controls who were selected from the same schools and who had had similar prodromal illnesses but had not developed Reye's syndrome. The questionnaire they administered was extensive; it sought information on seventy-three categories of possible exposure, residential and family history, personal medical history, immunizations, medications, characteristics of the prodromal illness, dietary history, and possible exposure to toxic products in the home or from animals. The interviews took place between four and eighty-three days after the onset of the children's illnesses; the average was six and a half weeks. Their hope was to identify one or more commonalities shared among the children who contracted Reye's syndrome that were not shared with the children in the control group.

In their initial study of twenty-five of the eighty-three children reported to have developed Reye's syndrome, Waldman and his colleagues found nine different categories of exposure that at least 80 percent of the children shared. For seven of the nine categories, there was no statistical difference between the children who had contracted Reye's syndrome and the children in the control group. "For two items, aspirin and vitamins," they reported, "there was a significant statistical difference between cases and controls." Of the children who had contracted RS, 84 percent had received regular vitamin supplements before their illness, but only 52 percent of their matched controls had. As for aspirin, 96 percent of the children with RS had received salicylate-containing products, compared with only 65 percent of the children in the control group. Waldman and his colleagues reported these data to the CDC, which, combined with Starko's paper and reports from Ohio, led to the article in *Morbidity and Mortality Weekly Report* late in 1980.

Recognizing both the tremendous potential of the three initial reports as well as their shortcomings, officials at the CDC pressed for better studies that would clarify a possible relationship between Reye's syndrome and aspirin. In response, the Michigan Department of Public Health hired Harry McGee and William Hall, both of whom had experience investigating disease outbreaks, to help Waldman conduct a second study in Michigan. Their study would focus directly on a possible link between RS and aspirin and be designed from the start to overcome the weaknesses of the previous three studies. What happened next was a turning point in the history of Reye's syndrome. At precisely the moment that researchers seemed on the verge of identifying a relationship between RS and aspirin, Reye's syndrome began to disappear—and disappear quickly.

Like me, Harry McGee now works at Michigan State University, and I have had the opportunity to talk with him about the Michigan studies several times. He described how, after working with Waldman on smallpox eradication in Bangladesh, he found himself working with him again in Michigan. McGee's deep respect for Waldman is apparent: "He's an amazing guy," McGee said, "a pillar in the international public health community." Together with William Hall and the state registrar, George Van Amburg, they began a second study in the winter of 1980–1981 that focused specifically on the possible relationship between Reye's syndrome and medications taken during a prodromal illness. They found, as researchers in every study after 1980 found, that it was increasingly difficult to find cases of Reye's syndrome to study. While the 1979–1980 winter had produced eighty-three cases in Michigan, the following year saw only eighteen.

The goal of the second study was to test the reproducibility of the most significant findings from the first study, to gather additional data, and to refine the study's methods to resolve some of the problems that had been identified with the first study. The investigators chose to exclude six of the eighteen children who had been given a diagnosis of Reye's syndrome because they were of preschool age and they could not identify comparable controls for children who did not have classmates. The questionnaire they used in the second study was much shorter, and it concentrated only on the medications that children received during the course of the illnesses. In contrast to the six-and-half-week average time between illnesses and interviews in the first study, McGee told me how the team had interviewed parents between two and ten days (on average, fewer than five days) after the onset of symptoms. After Waldman, Hall, and McGee had collected their data, Van Amburg did the statistical analysis. Thinking back on it, McGee said, "It amazes me to think that Van Amburg did all that with a simple calculator." They found that all twelve children who had contracted Reye's syndrome had received aspirin, compared to less than half of the children in the control group, and they failed to find anything to support the relationship between vitamins and RS that had been seen in the first study. Ultimately, their work provided the clearest evidence of a relationship between Reye's syndrome and aspirin. However, the relatively small number of cases of RS that year made the study less significant than they had hoped. Ironically, the decline in cases seemed both a blessing and a curse, as fewer children suffered the life-threatening ailment while researchers were left lacking the data they needed to better understand Reye's syndrome and its causes.

The Rise of the Aspirin Hypothesis

After reports emerged from the studies in Arizona, Ohio, and Michigan, the aspirin hypothesis quickly gained traction in both popular and professional venues. After a decade and a half of speculations and slow progress amid increasing public awareness (and fear) of Reye's syndrome, parents and physicians hoped an explanation was finally within sight. Over the previous decade, RS had been increasingly linked to influenza, so the flu season—which typically began in early winter and lasted until early spring—was heralded by a growing number of public service announcements reminding physicians and parents about the possibility that influenza sometimes turned into Reye's syndrome. By the early 1980s, the flu and Reye's syndrome were closely linked in the public's mind, especially in the Great Lakes region where Reye's syndrome was more common. For example, early in 1980 in the small farming community of Sherwood, Michigan, school officials shut down the town's elementary school after three children with influenza developed Reye's syndrome. Two of them died, and parents protested the scheduled reopening of the school a week later and complained about experts' inability to explain the illness. Mary Duttlinger, the mother of one of the two children who had died, expressed parents' frustration: "One doctor says do one thing. One doctor says another thing. People don't know what to do." The emergence later that year of evidence that a viral illness and aspirin might somehow combine to trigger Reye's syndrome was greeted with tremendous relief by many parents.

News that officials might have finally identified a cause that explained Reye's syndrome quickly found its way into the nation's major newspapers. The day after the CDC's *Morbidity and Mortality Weekly Report* published a preliminary description of the findings from Arizona, Ohio, and Michigan, the *New York Times* reported that researchers had completed two "large-scale, controlled studies of the relationship between Reye's syndrome and aspirin" and had found support for "suspicions that giving aspirin to children during a viral illness may encourage development of Reye's syndrome." Less than two months later, the *Washington Post* reported, "Its causes still are unknown, but recent studies have established a link between the incidence of Reye's syndrome and the use of medicines containing salicylates—simple aspirin." The *Post*'s article was republished in its entirety by the *Los Angeles Times* two weeks later. By March 1981, the American Academy of Pediatrics (AAP) Committee on Infectious Diseases and its Committee on Drugs reviewed the paper from Starko's team as well as initial reports from Ohio and Michigan, and they concluded that the research had "shown an association between the administration of aspirin to children with acute febrile illnesses, particularly influenza and varicella, and the subsequent development of Reye's syndrome."

The initial reports all concluded by emphasizing that much more research was needed before anyone could conclusively say that aspirin was linked to the development of Reye's syndrome, much less that it caused Reye's syndrome. Remember, for example, how the editors' note that accompanied the publication of the early findings in the *Morbidity and Mortality Weekly Report* in 1980 had identified several important shortcomings in the early studies and stressed that further analysis was needed. Likewise, in the *New York Times* article that was published the next day, Michael Gregg, the Deputy Director of the CDC's Bureau of Epidemiology pointed out that center officers were "not saying don't use aspirin. We are saying that there are studies that suggest that aspirin may be more associated with Reye syndrome than we would normally expect, and this implies a relationship between the two but it does not prove it." Given the intensity of the rhetoric that would emerge over the next several years—not to mention the triumphalist language that would be employed at the end of the century—these initial reports were quick to assert that even if aspirin were involved in the onset of Reye's syndrome, it could at most be part of the explanation for its cause. Take, for instance, the AAP's statement: "But even if aspirin is ultimately shown to play a role in the pathogenesis of Reye's syndrome, it cannot be the entire explanation, for the reason that the syndrome shows a particular predilection for individuals with influenza (particularly influenza B) and varicella and is much less frequent following other febrile illnesses of comparable severity." However, it is easy to understand why parents—who had grown increasingly frightened of Reye's syndrome over the previous decade and who regularly read reports of the deadly and mysterious ailment—were quick to accept that aspirin was the culprit, especially when they had other pain relievers and fever reducers to give their children.

When to Warn?

The EIS officers' findings in Arizona, Ohio, and Michigan were a significant breakthrough in the seventeen-year international effort to understand Reye's syndrome. Their work demonstrated a strong correlation between Reye's syndrome and aspirin by comparing children with minor illnesses who developed RS with other children who had similar illnesses but did not develop the much more serious symptoms of encephalitis and fatty degeneration of the viscera. The EIS officers and their colleagues in Arizona, Ohio, and Michigan found that the children who developed Reye's syndrome almost always took medications that contained salicylates, while their RS-free counterparts took fewer such products. Combined with the hints that had emerged over the previous two decades—stretching all the way back to the work done by Mortimer and Lepow in 1962—it seemed prudent to conclude that there was likely a relationship between Reye's syndrome and aspirin.

Aspirin consumption alone, however, could not explain the onset of Reye's syndrome, and no one in the early 1980s suggested that it did. It was clear from earlier studies that for the symptoms of Reye's syndrome to develop, aspirin consumption had to be combined with a viral infection of some sort. Even then, the vast majority of children that had such a viral infection and were treated with aspirin did not develop the characteristic symptoms of Reye's syndrome. Influenza B seemed to be the most common prodromal illness, but even today we lack solid scientific evidence to explain why. It was rare to find cases like mine in which there was either no identified prodromal illnesses or such a short period of time between the onset of a prodromal illness and the development of the much more serious symptoms of RS. One explanation for the necessity of a prodromal illness was Crocker's hypothesis, which suggested that exposure to toxins predisposed a child to be incapable of dealing with a typically routine viral infection. Another is a hypothesis that emerged in the late 1980s and was advanced by a number of former EIS officers that suggested that in children who developed Reye's syndrome, salicylate levels appeared to accumulate throughout the course of their prodromal illnesses. Either of these explanations required that aspirin consumption be combined with a viral illness, which is precisely what the evidence at hand suggested happened in almost all of the cases. Viral illnesses are inescapable, but children do not need to be given aspirin. So it was certainly reasonable to suggest to parents that they consider avoiding aspirin for children with viral illnesses.

Late in 1980, the CDC convened a working group of scientific consultants to evaluate the four studies that had come from Arizona, Ohio, and Michigan. In November 1981 they released a report concluding that, "there is strong epidemiologic evidence for an association between the occurrence of Reye's syndrome and prior ingestion of salicylate containing medication." The growing evidence of a correlation between aspirin and Reye's syndrome led the U.S. Department of Health and Human Services (HHS) and the CDC to issue a cautious joint statement in February 1982 "advising parents and physicians that the use of aspirin to treat children with chicken pox or flu-like illnesses has been linked with 'possible increased risk' of a life-threatening disease called Reye syndrome." The statement stopped short of telling parents not to give aspirin to children, but four months later two different authorities became much more assertive about warning parents of the relationship between RS and aspirin. First, in the June issue of their journal, *Pediatrics*, the American Academy of Pediatrics issued a carefully worded overview of the evidence suggesting a relationship between aspirin and RS and concluded "there is a high probability that the administration of aspirin contributes to the causation of Reye syndrome." That same month, Richard S. Schweiker, the secretary of the Department of Health and Human Services, informed the press that he had "directed the Surgeon General of the United States, Dr. C. Everett Koop, to issue the advisory and had also requested the Food and Drug Administration to require manufacturers of children's aspirin to put warning labels on their products and to conduct an appropriate education campaign aimed at doctors, pharmacists and parents." To that end, the HHS issued official notification to interested parties that would begin work on regulations that would require the labeling of aspirin bottles, an important step in the process that might eventually lead to warning labels on aspirin bottles—and one that incited considerable opposition.

Despite the published evidence from the EIS officers, the earlier work that coincided with it, careful articulation of a possible association between RS and aspirin, and the explanation of aspirin's potentially synergistic relationship with viral infections, there was significant opposition to the HHS's proposed rule that aspirin bottles be labeled. Not surprisingly, the aspirin manufacturers vigorously opposed it. In the early 1980s, the tremendous number of aspirin pills Americans consumed every year were the source of millions of dollars of profit for aspirin manufacturers. Already under increasing market pressure from acetaminophen and ibuprofen, the alleged connection to Reye's syndrome was deeply threatening to aspirin's market share. A handful of pediatricians expressed concern that the loss of aspirin as a tool for treating childhood fevers and pain would far outweigh any benefits gained from a possible decline in cases of Reye's syndrome. Aspirin's nearly century-long record of safety and efficacy, combined with the tremendous rarity of diagnosed cases of Reye's syndrome, motivated these physicians to resist public health officials' calls to stop giving aspirin to children suffering from viral illnesses. As earnest as some of them might have been in their criticisms of the aspirin hypothesis and their opposition to mandatory labeling, it is difficult to disentangle their public stance on the subject from the influence of the aspirin industry. The industry's deep pockets, aggressive legal tactics, and political patronage made it a powerful force in the political debates that emerged in the 1980s over Reye's syndrome and aspirin.

Public health officials scored two major victories early in 1982, with the American Academy of Pediatrics coming out in favor of the aspirin hypothesis and the secretary of the Department of Health and Human Services announcing plans to require that manufacturers label aspirin bottles with warnings about Reye's syndrome. However, those victories were short lived. Before the end of the year, advocates for the aspirin manufacturers had rolled back both of these victories and had established a political stalemate over the question of whether there was a relationship between aspirin and Reye's syndrome.

CHAPTER SIX

The Aspirin Industry Responds

Almost as soon as the Epidemic Intelligence Service officers developed the first evidence of a relationship between aspirin and Reye's syndrome, the companies that manufactured and sold aspirin resisted it. Their product had a century-old reputation for safety, and they responded to the aspirin hypothesis with calls for additional research and demands that regulators demonstrate a high level of certainty about a causal relationship—not merely a correlation—between aspirin and Reye's syndrome. Their reaction has become iconic of the kind of efforts put forward by industries to slow or avoid regulation. Over the last decade, the history of their efforts to discredit the aspirin hypothesis has become an example of industries' production and promotion of so-called junk science, but it had not originated with them. For example, in a 2005 article in the *American Journal of Public Health*, David Michaels and Celeste Monforton asserted, "The aspirin manufacturers did not invent the strategy of questioning the underlying science in order to prevent regulation; it had been successfully employed for decades by polluters and producers of hazardous products."

Throughout the summer and fall of 1982, representatives for the aspirin industry dealt serious setbacks to the successes that proponents of the aspirin hypothesis had achieved that spring when the American Academy of Pediatrics (AAP) and the U.S. Department of Health and Human Services (HHS) approved the claim that there might be a relationship between aspirin and Reye's syndrome. On the heels of the HHS announcement in April that the department would start an educational campaign about the possible relationship between aspirin and RS and take under consideration a requirement to label aspirin bottles, a spokesman for the company that manufactured Bayer aspirin claimed that the warnings were "inappropriate." According to him, "There is no scientific basis for a causal association between aspirin and the development of Reye's Syndrome. We are confident the company will be able to convince [HHS] Secretary Schweiker and the commissioner [of the Food and Drug Administration] to re-review the matter."

In April 1982, just as the AAP and the HHS were beginning to publicize their assessments that there appeared to be a relationship between aspirin and Reye's syndrome, a group of aspirin manufactures formed the Aspirin Foundation of America. Funded primarily by Bayer, one of the world's largest aspirin manufacturers, the Aspirin Foundation was launched at a symposium at the Tulane University School of Medicine. Eighteen medical authorities presented papers at the conference, which was designed to showcase aspirin's safety and its efficacy in reducing pain and fever. Cochaired by G. Gilbert McMahon and Louis Lasagna—who coincidentally were members of the Congressional Commission on the Federal Drug Approval Process—the conference hosted papers lauding aspirin's usefulness. "This remarkable analgesic drug remains unappreciated by many physicians," McMahon declared.

Joseph White, the first president of the newly founded Aspirin Foundation, quickly became the leading voice in efforts to undermine the aspirin hypothesis and stall efforts to label aspirin bottles with warnings about Reye's syndrome. The aspirin industry could not have invented a better advocate. Even his name was perfect for the task: St. Joseph was the name of a popular children's aspirin, and white is a color generally associated with aspirin and medicine. A physician, White was quoted in most of the newspaper reports on the subject throughout the early 1980s and was always harshly critical of claims of any relationship—much less a causal one—between aspirin and Reye's syndrome. Early in the summer of 1982, just after the HHS reported that it would begin an educational campaign and consider labeling aspirin bottles, White and the Aspirin Foundation launched a media blitz to discredit the aspirin hypothesis. In a *Washington Post* story he announced that his group would consider filing a lawsuit to block the labeling requirement. "White said that the studies linking aspirin use to the syndrome 'were so faulty and poorly run they couldn't be subjected to valid statistical analysis. . . . The evidence doesn't warrant this step.'" Similarly, White was quoted in the *New York Times* three days later saying that the four state studies were "wholly inconclusive" and that the HHS "acted hastily and without scientific basis." White's claims were widely publicized, appearing in newspapers across the country throughout the summer.

The clearest articulation of the Aspirin Foundation's argument came in July with the publication of a long letter to the editor of *Pediatrics*. Titled "Reye Syndrome and Salicylates: A Spurious Association" and published under the byline "RS Working Group," the letter asserted that the shortcomings of the case-control studies in Arizona, Ohio, and Michigan made "all inferences pertaining to association or causality between aspirin and RS highly questionable—or worse—misleading." The letter identified three major criticisms of the research that had led CDC and HHS officials to believe that there might be a causal relationship between RS and aspirin. First, it attacked the methods used for selecting both cases and controls, and it focused special attention on the Ohio study. Given that the Ohio study was originally designed to investigate the prodromal illnesses the preceded the onset of Reye's syndrome and was later directed at the question of the role of aspirin, it was relatively easy to argue that the study was ill suited to demonstrating aspirin's involvement. Second, the letter asserted biases in the collection of data, especially as it related to parents' confusion of aspirin with acetaminophen and their tendency to misremember details of their children's illnesses. Finally, it argued that recent laboratory and clinical data suggested that there was little biological plausibility of a causal association between aspirin and RS. Ultimately, the RS Working Group concluded, "The only responsible statement[s] that can be made in relation to RS at this time are those that pertain to *early recognition of RS* and to *prudent use of all medications* [emphasis in the original]."

The Aspirin Foundation of America still exists and now is funded exclusively by the German pharmaceutical company Bayer Healthcare and the British company Reckitt Benckiser, whose brands include a large number of household cleaners and over-the-counter drugs. The foundation's website still includes a long statement about its position on the alleged relationship between aspirin and Reye's syndrome. Today, even after warning labels have been on aspirin bottles for more than a quarter of a century, Reye's syndrome has disappeared, and the aspirin hypothesis is nearly universally accepted, the Aspirin Foundation asserts that "the evidence behind this association is far from conclusive and the restrictions on using aspirin have long been controversial."

Sometime in 1982, a second organization funded by a pharmaceutical company, the Committee for the Care of Children, emerged and argued against the aspirin hypothesis as well as the associated effort to label aspirin bottles with warnings about Reye's syndrome. Schering-Plough and Sterling Drug, which manufactured St. Joseph's Aspirin for children, funded the Boston-based organization. In November 1982, the Committee on the Care of Children filed an unsuccessful action in federal district court to stop HHS secretary Schweiker's public service campaign about the possible link between aspirin and RS.

A third pro-aspirin industry organization also appeared, presenting itself as representing concerned parents. The American Reye's Syndrome Foundation (not to be confused with the National Reye's Syndrome Foundation) was based in Denver, Colorado. Throughout the early 1980s, as almost all the local and state chapters of Reye's syndrome advocacy organizations merged into the National Reye's Syndrome Foundation, the American Reye's Syndrome Foundation remained independent. John Freudenberger, one of the founders of the NRSF, stated that the American Reye's Syndrome Foundation had "always yielded to the Aspirin Foundation," adopting the industry's position that there should be no labeling of aspirin to warn of its potential link with RS. He believed that the American Reye's Syndrome Foundation needed "the money of the Aspirin Foundation" to survive and therefore parroted the industry's position on the issue of labeling.

The aspirin industry–funded organizations provided the media with easily quotable sound bites that undermined claims made by proponents of the aspirin hypothesis while at the same time they helped direct a growing movement inside Washington to avoid labeling aspirin bottles. Publicly, their representatives claimed to have been motivated by a sincere interest in upholding high standards of scientific rigor. Take, for example, the conclusion of the penultimate paragraph of the letter to the editor of *Pediatrics* from the Aspirin Foundation's RS Working Group: "In summary, examination of epidemiologic standards as they apply to appropriate RS survey data show that cases and controls represent different populations at base line in terms of nature and severity of illness and thus cannot be compared relative to aspirin usage. Any inferences from the survey should be used to refine the methodology and provide input to the design of future surveys that are based on scientifically sound principles."

While aspirin industry's representatives claimed to be pressing for high standards of scientific rigor, behind the scenes they were part of an effort that was intricately linked to a growing movement in Washington. The aspirin industry's interest in delaying or preventing the labeling of aspirin bottles with warnings about Reye's syndrome coincided with a growing movement to undermine the regulatory powers of federal agencies and departments like the Department of Health and Human Services.

The First House Hearings on Aspirin and Reye's Syndrome

In September 1982, as the nation's children returned to school from summer vacation and after months of lobbying from representatives of the aspirin industry, U.S. Representative James Scheuer called to order a two-day hearing on the alleged association between Reye's syndrome and aspirin. Scheuer was a liberal Democrat from New York and chairman of the Committee on Science and Technology's Subcommittee on Natural Resources, Agriculture Research, and Environment. In his opening statement, Scheuer made clear his interest in the controversy surrounding the alleged association of Reye's syndrome and the use of aspirin. He admitted that the issue was "somewhat emotionally charged, because the question of the health of our children is a very emotional commitment that most of us have," and thus he wanted to "proceed with great caution and do everything possible to assure their well-being." As the parent of four children, Scheuer described the agony he felt whenever his children were ill with even a benign illness, and he asserted the tremendous importance of "adequate guidance" from the government in treating children's illnesses. No medication, he said, has been used longer than aspirin. "It is a staple in everyone's medicine cabinet." Scheuer explained that both he and his children had long relied on aspirin to help them through life's inevitable illnesses and injuries.

From the start, the organization and conduct of the hearings made it clear that Scheuer intended to be highly critical of the decision by the Department of Health and Human Services to launch a campaign to warn parents about the alleged link between aspirin and Reye's syndrome. The testimony offered by the invited speakers constructed, step by step, a rejection of the evidence that suggested any connection as well as a condemnation of the HHS for warning parents of the supposed link. As such, it provided a highly visible showcase for the aspirin industry's refutation of the claim of any link between their product and Reye's syndrome.

The hearing opened with a formal statement from George Johnson, the lead author on the 1963 article describing the first identified cases of Reye's syndrome in the United States. By the 1980s, Johnson was a pediatrician practicing in Fargo, North Dakota, and a professor at the University of North Dakota. Scheuer asked him to provide a summary of the origins of Reye's syndrome and the efforts to identify its cause. Johnson described how, twenty years earlier, he had been a "young epidemiologist at the North Carolina State Health Department" when he received reports of sixteen cases of sudden death in young children coincident with an influenza B epidemic in the state. He gave a dramatic account of the first reported death of a child in the United States from Reye's syndrome and stated, "I believed at that time and I still do believe that we dealt with a new disease." His group was the first to associate RS with outbreaks of influenza, and he explained that it was later realized that about 10 percent of the cases of Reye's syndrome follow other illnesses, including varicella, parainfluenza, Coxsackievirus, adenovirus, and infectious mononucleosis. He also mentioned Crocker's work in Nova Scotia that linked RS to an emulsifier in the spray used to control the spruce budworm and described other ailments that induced symptoms similar to Reye's syndrome, including fungal toxins and Jamaican vomiting sickness.

Scheuer politely interrupted Johnson's testimony to ask for more details after Johnson brought up the relatively recent assertion that aspirin might be a factor in the development of the disease. Johnson said that he was not capable of providing the subcommittee with an expert judgment of the claim that aspirin might be causally linked to Reye's syndrome because he had "not been privy to the raw data." Instead, he offered his opinion based on his work in a group of twelve busy pediatricians in an active regional medical center in Fargo: "[W]e can say only that none of us has seen clinical association as general practicing pediatricians between Reye's syndrome and the ingestion of aspirin." With the recent efforts to educate parents about the possible threat posed by aspirin, he said that he and his colleagues had been deluged by phone calls and queries from parents. In effect, he testified, a warning against the use of aspirin in children with influenza was a warning against the use of aspirin in any child and at any time. It effectively eliminated aspirin as a useful weapon in pediatricians' and parents' arsenals.

For Johnson, the question of the alleged relationship between aspirin and Reye's syndrome was far from settled. He recounted the discussions that had appeared in the June 1982 issue of *Pediatrics* and asserted that "the Arizona, Michigan, and particularly the Ohio studies making the relationship [between aspirin and RS] have been strongly criticized because of lack of careful matching of the severity of the prodromal illness in both the cases and the controls." Johnson was particularly critical of studies that relied on parents' recall of the medications they gave their children as many as ten or twelve days earlier. In addition to the shortcomings in parents' memories, he said, people frequently used the term "aspirin" in reference to products containing salicylates, ibuprofen, or acetaminophen. His personal experience in private practice corroborated studies that suggested that up to 25 percent of parents inaccurately recalled the names of the over-the-counter drugs they had recently given their children. Johnson also expressed concern that the published studies had failed to ascertain the nature of the illnesses that children had suffered before their RS was diagnosed, which further undermined his confidence that the researchers were accurately comparing the rates of

RS diagnoses in children who had and had not received aspirin during the course of a bout of influenza.

Johnson's claim that his greatest concern was that by too easily adopting the hypothesis that aspirin caused Reye's syndrome, parent's and physicians would be lulled into a sense of complacency about RS and critical questions would not be pursued. He asked, "Will the clamor given this tenuous association divert the public and indeed divert practicing physicians from the urgent tasks of future research regarding this puzzling entity? Will they assume that the answer has been found, that there is an association between aspirin and Reye's syndrome?" Johnson repeated some of the pressing questions about aspirin and RS that had already been raised by both advocates and detractors of the aspirin hypothesis, including the need for research that would explain the seasonal incidence and geographical clustering of cases. He called for a better understanding of the typical course of Reye's syndrome, screening tests, improved treatments and reporting, and research on the long-term prognosis for children who survive a bout with it. "As a general practitioner of pediatrics," he concluded, "it is my opinion that we have invoked the jury before thoroughly evaluating all the evidence of Reye's syndrome."

Scheuer followed Johnson's prepared remarks with several questions, all of which focused on the impact of the Department of Health and Human Services' efforts to dissuade parents from giving aspirin to their children. Johnson expressed his amazement at the efficacy of the television ad campaign alleging a link between Reye's syndrome and aspirin and the speed at which the public had begun using less aspirin, which he believed was a safe and effective over-the-counter medication. He discussed his fear that parents would increase their use of acetaminophen, which would result in a larger number of acute poisonings, and he reiterated his concerns that the publicity around the alleged link between aspirin and RS would "divert us from the needs of Reye's syndrome in the future." He asserted that he was not alone in believing that "there is nothing to this business of aspirin and Reye's syndrome. . . . And again, it is an unscientific statement, but I have yet to talk to one of my conferees in pediatrics that does not agree."

After Johnson's testimony concluded, Scheuer introduced Heinz Eichenwald, a professor retired from the University of Texas Health Services Center, who continued the criticism of the HHS's decision to warn parents about a possible connection between Reye's syndrome and aspirin. Eichenwald was particularly critical of the methodological shortcomings he identified with the studies that led the HHS to issue their warnings, especially the second Ohio study. There was no specific diagnostic test for RS, so accurate diagnoses required a well-trained physician who could evaluate the available evidence and assess a series of probabilities to judge whether or not a child did indeed have Reye's syndrome. Among the most valuable tests was a liver biopsy, "an invasive and often painful procedure, which many physicians may not wish to perform." Eigenwald asserted that even with all of the available evidence at hand, "about 25 percent of the children who are sent to us [at Children's Medical Center of Dallas] from other hospitals for the diagnosis of Reye's syndrome turn out not to have it." He therefore discounted any of the studies that reported on the frequency of aspirin use in children that supposedly had Reye's syndrome because in his experience about one in four of the children did not actually suffer from RS. Moreover, in the reported studies of Reye's, Eichenwald saw that there were several symptoms suffered by children in the studies that did not conform to what he knew to be true about RS. The reported rates of the syndrome in the Ohio study were eight to twelve times higher than they had ever been, and the mortality rates were exceedingly low compared with previous reports. Finally, among the reported cases, there were many more children who suffered from the early stages of Reye's syndrome as compared to the numbers of children who suffered from advanced stages, and 80 percent of the children in the study never had a liver biopsy that would allow physicians to confirm their diagnoses.

Unlike Johnson, Eichenwald had recently had the opportunity to see the raw data on which the Ohio study was produced. After examining the case report forms that were submitted by the Ohio Department of Health, Eichenwald found that a number of the children had received inaccurate diagnoses and were not in fact suffering from Reye's syndrome. The investigators had relied upon blood tests, the results of which would have been similar in cases of Reye's syndrome and in cases in which children suffered from mild to moderate viral infections but not Reye's. A number of other children were never tested for elevated serum levels, which are indicative of RS. He concluded, "The patterns, the diagnoses, were simply not correct or could not be looked upon with a great deal of assurance."

Eichenwald had access to the data because he, along with five other pediatricians—Sidney Gellis, Robert Hoekelman, Philip Lanzkowsky, Henry Nadler, and Irving Shulman—had been given the information by Glenbrook Laboratories, a pharmaceutical company that produced aspirin for Bayer. Glenbrook's parent company, Sterling Drug, and the pharmaceutical company Schering-Plough had filed a Freedom of Information Act lawsuit to obtain the data, and the companies had asked the six pediatricians to review the data and make recommendations about what they believed was the best course of action based on their interpretations of the material. After reviewing the data, the group sent a telegram to the secretary of the Department of Health and Human Services: "We are disturbed to learn that the raw data were never analyzed by independent agencies until recently. This lack of analysis of raw data was a serious gap in the scientific process." They asserted that many of the afflicted children had actually not been given aspirin, and they called on the secretary to conduct a review of the data and its associated conclusions. "Any labeling," they warned, "should be delayed until such a review is completed. Labeling aspirin to warn against its use in influenza and chickenpox may be a premature activity. It may have public health consequences far more serious than the intent it has to cure."

In the question-and-answer period that followed Eichenwald's prepared statement, Scheuer contrasted the six hundred to a thousand cases of Reye's syndrome in the United States against the 150,000 American children who relied on aspirin to control the symptoms associated with juvenile arthritis. Aspirin was, according to Eichenwald, "the best antipyretic, antifever medicine that we have," and if the FDA decides to apply a warning label to it, "pediatrician[s] would be very reluctant to recommend [aspirin] because of the possibility of a malpractice suit if something should happen." Instead of wasting valuable resources convincing the public that aspirin was possibly dangerous to children, Scheur and Eichenwald both believed that the government should invest those resources into helping parents "be on the lookout for early warning signals of Reye's syndrome." It was simply bad science, Eichenwald stated, to accept the researchers' claims without a thorough evaluation of the raw data from which they worked, as well as all associated data. The CDC had not seen the raw data. "I am convinced," he concluded, "that if they had seen the data they would have arrived at the same conclusion that these six prominent pediatrics professors did who had seen it at the time."

The testimony offered by Robert Klein, director of the Dartmouth-Hitchcock Arthritis Center, furthered the argument that warnings about a possible link between aspirin and Reye's syndrome would ultimately eliminate aspirin as one of the tools pediatricians could use in treating sick children. Aspirin was critical to the treatment of children with rheumatoid arthritis, and researchers and clinicians associated with the disease were concerned that premature warnings against the use of aspirin in children would eliminate aspirin as a therapeutic tool against juvenile arthritis. Klein's center had polled clinicians from the United States, South America, and England who specialized in juvenile arthritis, asking about the incidence of Reye's syndrome in their patients "We find," he reported, that there are a handful of cases of Reye's syndrome but not the increased incidence apparently one would expect to see." As a result of the HHS's warnings about the alleged link between aspirin and RS, he explained, "many of us are receiving phone calls from patients about the fear of the use of aspirin. . . . We find ourselves really having trouble trying to get people to take aspirin."

Paul Hinson, the executive director of the Denver-based, industry-funded American Reye's Syndrome Association, took the stand and expressed his agreement with much of what Johnson, Eichwald, and Klein had already said. Even more forcefully than those who preceded him, Hinson explained that Reye's syndrome was still a "medical mystery" and was often fatal even though it had been aggressively researched. "There is no known cause," he said, "and the mechanism of the disease is not understood. We have at our disposal neither a cure nor any dependable means of prevention at this time." Like Johnson, he was concerned that media coverage of the alleged link between aspirin and Reye's syndrome would lull parents into a false sense of security. Efforts should be made toward increased awareness of the ailment and early detection, which is the "best preventative tool we have in hand."

The testimonies critical of the decision to warn parents about possible links between aspirin and Reye's syndrome concluded with an appearance before the subcommittee by Frank Hurley, president of the Biometric Research Institute in Arlington, Virginia. Hurley's company had been retained by Sterling Drug and Schering-Plough earlier that year to conduct an independent analysis of the raw data from the Ohio study that the companies had forced the Ohio Department of Health and the CDC to release. Schering-Plough had made repeated requests for the raw data beginning in November 1980 but did not have access to it until June 1982. Even then, Hurley asserted, he had not had access to all the raw data or the case histories from the Ohio study. Ultimately, from the evidence that was made available to him, Hurley concluded that the results of the Ohio studies "do not provide sound statistical evidence of any association between salicylate use and Reye's syndrome." His criticisms of the study repeated many of the criticisms offered by previous witnesses before the subcommittee.

Other than the first four witnesses—Johnson, Eichenwald, Klein, and Hurley—and Scheuer and majority counsel Jonah Shacknai, the only other voice that appears in the transcript to this point in the hearing was that of Maryanne C. Bach, the minority counsel. Bach briefly and respectfully probed each witness's assumptions about precisely when, where, and how he thought it would be appropriate for a government agency to offer a warning about a potential adverse effect from unregulated over-the-counter medication. "At what point," she asked, "should the agency say something and not be accused of withholding information? On the other hand, how does the agency avoid unnecessary paranoia about something?" All the witnesses seemed to agree that an agency is justified in issuing such a warning only after appropriate professionals from outside the government have examined the issue and rendered their advice.

The first four witnesses provided several hours of detailed testimony that was critical of the HHS's decision to—in their depiction of the situation—accept uncritically the findings of the second Ohio study and issue a warning directly to parents. Their testimony was followed by polite and encouraging questions from Scheuer and Shacknai, who helped sharpen some of the witnesses' claims and made even harsher some of their criticisms of the HHS.

The first witness to offer at least some support for the HHS's decision to issue a warning to parents about possible links between aspirin and Reye's syndrome was John Crocker, the professor of epidemiology from Dalhousie University, who had investigated claims in the early 1970s that Reye's syndrome might be linked to the spraying against spruce budworm. Crocker believed that "a plethora of chemicals and agents" had been linked to Reye's syndrome, including "latex paints, aflatoxin, a series of chemical connections, [with] aspirin being one of them." It is difficult to avoid thinking that Crocker's support for the aspirin hypothesis—lukewarm as it was—had something to do with Scheuer's admonition to him to be as brief as possible with his testimony. After allowing Johnson, Eichenwald, Klein, and Hurley unlimited time for their testimonies, Scheuer instructed Crocker to provide a statement and a reflection on prior testimonies "in 10 minutes to the second."

Unlike the previous witnesses, who had been uniformly inclined to give aspirin the benefit of the doubt until significant evidence against it emerged, Crocker admitted that he was "not certain that aspirin has a complete clear bill of health." Ultimately, he believed that some children might be inclined to develop the symptoms that are associated with Reye's syndrome and taking "aspirin may slant the curve." That is, Crocker believed that aspirin's effects on already stressed bodies could trigger RS. He said that he believed that "Reye's syndrome is multifactorial and there may be a different set of chemicals involved with varicella and different with influenza, and that may account for the regional differences." Crocker was not forceful in his criticism of the HHS's decision to issue a warning on aspirin, but he concluded by saying, "Really, I think the warning label rather than warning physicians may have been a bit of overkill."

The next witness, Reule Stallones, dean of the School of Public

Health at the University of Texas in Houston, pulled the microphone toward himself and announced, "I have begun to suspect that I am a minority in this assemblance [sic] this morning, which I trust will be a spiritually salutary experience for me." Stallones had been the cochairman of the meeting on Reye's syndrome held earlier that year at Johns Hopkins University that was sponsored by the CDC and the NIH. He reported that at the meeting "the full array of opinions possible was expressed, from firm belief that the use of salicylates in the treatment of influenza, chickenpox, and other viral infections is directly a cause of Reye's syndrome to the opinion that salicylates are valuable and virtually innocuous drugs whose use should not be curtailed to any degree." Most participants, he said, took some intermediate view between these two extremes. The participants examined the four epidemiologic studies of the Reye's syndrome, one each from Arizona and Ohio and two from Michigan, and Stallones asserted, "In all of the studies the proportion of cases of Reye's syndrome found to have used salicylates prior to their illness was in excess of 95 percent. The proportion of salicylate users among the noncases was much lower than that, ranging generally perhaps to around 50 percent."

Stallones reported that there were only four possible explanations for the notable difference in salicylate consumption among the children who had developed Reye's syndrome and those who had not. One, it was possible that the significant difference was merely a chance occurrence, but the chances of this happening were very small—one or two in a thousand—so this was an unlikely explanation. Two, the findings could be the result of bias in the studies, especially if there was a strong tendency to overstate the use of salicylates in cases of Reye's syndrome and understate it in noncases. Several methods of analysis were applied to the results that strongly suggested that such a bias would have not resulted in the findings that emerged from all four studies. Three, the association could have been the result of the fact that the children who suffered from Reye's had required a great deal more medical intervention than had the children whose illnesses never developed the symptoms associated with RS. Therefore, the children with Reye's syndrome would likely have received more salicylates than did the children who did not develop

RS. To rule out this possibility, the researchers compared rates of salicylate use among children who suffered illnesses to a similar degree, and they still found differences in the rates of salicylate use between cases and noncases of RS. Four—and the only explanation that held up after the others had been examined—was that there was "some causal link between salicylate usage and occurrence of Reye's syndrome." But that does not, he concluded, mean that aspirin is necessarily the only factor involved in inducing Reye's syndrome.

As a result of the analysis of the four studies in Arizona, Ohio, and Michigan, Stallones believed that the "minimum acceptable response to the problem" was to warn physicians and parents of the possible hazards of giving aspirin to children suffering from viral illnesses. He stated his belief that "salicylates are used much too freely in the treatment of children with modestly elevated temperatures and that reduction of that use, especially for children with influenza and chickenpox, would carry no penalty at all." He concluded by asserting—in sharp contrast to the witnesses who preceded him—that "we have sufficient information that salicylates may pose a hazard . . . [and] to do nothing appears to me to be irresponsible."

While a subtle change in Scheuer's and Shacknai's demeanor had preceded Crocker's testimony, their treatment of Stallones differed radically from the cooperative, polite treatment that Johnson, Eichenwald, Klein, and Hurley had received. After Stallones finished his short statement, Scheuer thanked him and asked if he had seen the raw data from the studies. Stallones had not seen it, and as he tried to say that the raw data ought to be analyzed, Scheuer twice cut him off and asserted that without "scrutiny of the entire medical community" political decisions would be made based on research that "may be fatally flawed." Stallones agreed and tried to elaborate, but Scheuer again cut him off abruptly and preached about the need for good, open, and carefully studied scientific conclusions to form the basis for good policy before handing the floor over to Shacknai, subcommittee's majority counsel.

Shacknai probed Stallones' claims about the breadth of support among scientists of a causal link between aspirin and Reye's syndrome. Stallones had asserted that "several prestigious groups" had supported his conclusions, but on questioning it appeared that only the CDC working group on Reye's syndrome had produced the conclusions and two other groups—an FDA working group and an NIH consensus panel—did not issue a statement that it had found there was a link between Reye's and aspirin. Instead, they merely reported that the CDC working group had decided that there might be a causal relationship. The day's testimony concluded in time for the participants to have a late lunch, and it took another twelve days before members of the subcommittee met again to conclude the hearing.

In Defense of the Ohio Study

On September 29, 1982, Scheur was joined by Rep. Claudine Schneider, a Republican from Rhode Island, and the minority and majority counsels, Shacknai and Bach, to complete testimony on the alleged association between Reye's syndrome and aspirin. The minutes did not record which members were present at the first half of the hearing, and Scheuer, Shacknai, and Bach's were the only voices recorded in the transcript.

Scheuer opened the second day of the hearing with a bold pronouncement: based on the testimony the subcommittee had already heard, he said, "the evidence that there is some kind of cause and effect between ingesting aspirin and developing Reye's syndrome is far too tentative and far too flawed for any type of regulatory action to be contemplated." He was, therefore, "especially concerned" to learn that Richard Schweiker, secretary of the Department of Health and Human Services, had announced only days earlier that his department "was going ahead with a public education program against aspirin use as well as with labeling changes on aspirin bottles." In light of this, Scheuer was happy to announce that the day's first witness would be Edward Brandt, the assistant secretary for health in the Department of Health and Human Services. He was accompanied by Harry Meyer, the director of the National Center for Drugs and Biologics at the Food and Drug Administration; Walter Dowdle, the director of the Center for Infectious Diseases at the Centers for Disease Control; Gerald Quinnan, the director of the Division of Virology at the National Center for Drugs and Biologics; and Eugene Hurwitz, a physician and CDC employee who helped design and oversee the much maligned second Ohio study and who would eventually lead a major study on the relationship between RS and medications from 1984 through 1986 for the U.S. Public Health Service.

Brandt, fully aware that he was in hostile territory, began by summarizing the statement he had submitted that described the scientific evidence linking aspirin and Reye's syndrome and outlining the Department of Health and Human Services's efforts to inform the public of the possible link. "The association," he asserted, "is not new. A number of investigators over the past twenty years have suggested that Reye's syndrome may be associated with salicylates." He recounted how, two years earlier, studies in Arizona, Ohio, and Michigan had provided evidence to support the hypothesis that there was a relationship between aspirin and RS. In November 1980, the studies had led the CDC to issue a warning: "Parents should be advised to use caution when administering salicylates to treat children with viral illnesses, particularly chickenpox and influenza-like illnesses." A year later the CDC convened the meeting at Johns Hopkins University of "outside experts" that Stallones had already described, which concluded that there was "strong epidemiologic evidence for an association between the occurrence of Reye's syndrome and the prior ingestion of salicylate-containing medication." Two months later, the CDC released another warning to physicians and parents about the possibility of a causal association. In response to the CDC's warnings, the Food and Drug Administration formed their working group from members of the agency to review the available data, which released its report in May 1982. That same month the CDC, FDA, and the NIH—the nation's three most influential government agencies on matters related to health and medicine—had convened the meeting at Johns Hopkins University.

Brandt explained that, based on the scientific studies and associated reviews by scientific and government authorities over the previous two years, Secretary Schweiker of the HHS had just announced a proposal to label all over-the-counter, nonprescription drugs that contained salicylates. Coming during the time between the first and second halves of the hearing, Schweiker's announcement surely would have irritated Scheuer and Shacknai. The proposed label would read: "Warning: This product contains salicylate. Do not use in persons under 16 years of age with flu or chickenpox unless directed by your doctor. The use of salicylates to treat these conditions has been reported to be associated with a rare but serious childhood illness called Reye's syndrome." In conjunction with this new warning would be an HHS-sponsored public awareness campaign that would include radio public service announcements and brochures for doctors to provide to patients and parents. Brandt concluded by quoting a statement Stallones made at the end of his testimony twelve days earlier: "Taking action on evidence that is incomplete or inconclusive is commonly required, and the decision to do so is usually uncomfortable and sometimes agonizing. However, in this instance we have sufficient information that salicylate may pose a hazard that to do nothing appears to me to be irresponsible."

In the question-and-answer period that followed Brandt's statement, Scheuer pursued only one question: did the scientific and government authorities who proclaimed a causal link between Reye's syndrome and aspirin have direct access to the raw data on which the Ohio study was based? Walter Dowdle, director of the CDC's Center for Infectious Diseases, was the first to address Scheuer's questions, but he quickly turned to Eugene Hurwitz, the CDC employee who had been part of the second Ohio study. Scheuer asked him whether he had direct access to the data over and over again and in a number of different ways. Hurwitz was steadfast. Yes, he had seen the raw data. Yes, he had worked directly with the data. Yes, he was and he remained satisfied with the scientific validity of the raw data. After having Hurwitz on record as stating that throughout the investigation and write up of the report, he had access to and had seen the raw data, Scheuer turned the floor over to Shacknai.

Shacknai had in hand a stack of letters from earlier that year that he claimed had "fallen into the hands of the subcommittee" and detailed the CDC's complaints about a "lack of access to the raw data, specifically the individual questionnaires used in the four case-control studies." The letters were written by a variety of people, including the CDC's legal advisor, a contracting and procurement officer for the CDC, and Thomas Halpin, the project's chief investigator. The researchers in Ohio had refused to release the contents of the questionnaires because the results of the studies had not yet been published. With Hurwitz on record as having firmly stated that he had unfettered access to the raw data and had analyzed it carefully, Shacknai declared that "every piece of correspondence" and Thomas Halpin's deposition "would indicate that in fact neither members of the CDC team nor members of any other Federal Government team did in fact have access to the raw data really at any point until the FDA group came in and did its preliminary review, and even then they were not permitted to remove such data from the premises, nor to make photographic reproductions of such data." The revelation had all the makings of a courtroom gotcha moment as Shacknai sprang the trap that Rep. Scheuer had set.

For the next several minutes, Scheuer pressed the five men for more details about who had access to the raw data, when, and to what degree they evaluated the validity of the data. With almost every new question came a new respondent, as the witnesses shuffled to put the most authoritative voice in front of the microphone. As a result, Scheuer made little headway in pressing his argument that the scientific analyses—and thus the policies that resulted from them—were based on weak or faulty data. In response, Brandt and his colleagues tried to steer the conversation away from issues related to the quality of the data and toward discussion of the difference between causal relationships and correlations. At one point, Harry Meyer, director of the National Center for Drugs and Biologics at the FDA, seized control of the conversation and asserted to Scheuer, "You keep using the term 'cause-and-effect relationship.' No one feels that the data show a cause-and-effect relationship. The people feel, though, no matter how hard we critically analyze[d] the data . . . we were left with a strong association, but an association, not a cause-and-effect relationship."

Scheuer and Shacknai responded by abandoning the critique of the studies themselves to focus on the nature of the warning that there appeared to be an association between aspirin and Reye's syndrome. Brandt asserted that, based on the research, officials faced the question, "[A]t what point do you alert the physicians?" Scheuer quickly responded, "You see, we would have no question at all if you had gone to the physicians, because physicians can fine tune their approach . . . But when you go beyond the physicians and over the heads of physicians to the mothers of America and you advise them not to use aspirin for a very small group of kids, what we are afraid of, as you undoubtedly know by now is that somehow or other in the fuzzy business of communicating, mothers will interpret this warning as a warning that aspirin is bad, aspirin is dangerous, and that if you take aspirin, your child may get Reye's syndrome." Brandt explained that officials had already gone to the physicians two years earlier with warnings of a possible association between aspirin and Reye's syndrome, and that "most physicians are used to dealing with the issue of competing risks in managing patients."

It would seem at first blush that Scheuer and presumably Shacknai were principally concerned that the HHS's warnings about aspirin and Reye's syndrome would undermine the authority of the physicians, who were best able to weigh the risks in treating individual patients. However, Scheuer bluntly stated, "Don't you understand, Dr. Brandt, we are not concerned with physicians." Instead, he was worried that the "fuzzy" warning the HHS offered to parents would result in a stigma on aspirin. "Really, this is the only problem we are talking about," he explained, "not whether an advisory would not have been totally appropriate to physicians." Brandt attempted to reassure Scheuer that the department would "be as cautious as humanly possible" to make their message to parents clear, but Scheuer cut him off. "How about the danger of malpractice suits? I can see physicians being afraid to prescribe aspirin now," he said.

Scheuer and Shacknai spent the better part of the next hour grilling the five witnesses about the makeup of the review panels, the quality and availability of the evidence produced by the second Ohio study, and criticisms of the alleged association between aspirin and Reye's syndrome. As with their earlier efforts to describe the differences between a causal relationship and a correlation, the witnesses nudged Scheuer's and Shacknai's questions about data quality into a conversation about the norms of scientific investigations, the nature of open-ended scientific investigations, and the researchers' efforts to uncover some of the factors that appeared to be involved in the onset of Reye's syndrome. Their testimony ended with a promise from Brandt that they would "walk cautiously" through the minefield of the alleged association between Reye's syndrome and aspirin. Scheuer replied, "What we want you to do is stand instead of walk."

The hearing's last witness allowed Scheuer and Shacknai to close with yet another set of attacks on the alleged association between aspirin and Reye's syndrome. They called to the witness table James Orlowski, the assistant director of pediatrics in the intensive care unit of the Rainbow Babies and Children's Hospital in Cleveland, Ohio. Orlowski specialized in the treatment of critically ill children, had treated about twenty children with Reye's syndrome, and had worked directly with R. D. K. Reye in the Royal Alexandra Hospital for Sick Children in Sydney. Some of the records from the patients he had treated had become part of the second Ohio study, and he was concerned that cases he had reported were excluded from the study. His analysis of the published data suggested that there was significant selection bias in the study because, as it appeared to him, a disproportionate number of the children who had developed RS but had not ingested aspirin were excluded from the analysis. Moreover the very low death rate of children in the study who were reported as suffering from Reye's syndrome—which was only about 5 percent—was much lower than the 20 percent to 30 percent mortality expected in children who actually had Reye's syndrome. Much of Orlowski's testimony repeated what witnesses had stated on the first day of the hearing: the studies suffered from a number of methodological errors and, while there might be some association between aspirin and Reye's syndrome, there was far too little solid evidence linking the two to recommend eliminating a valuable medication for childhood illnesses and injuries.

Orlowski was an excellent witness to call at the close of the hearing because he was so forceful in his attack on the HHS's warnings to parents about the alleged dangers of aspirin. He stated that, from his experience with childhood pain-relievers and fever-reducers, "acetaminophen is a much more dangerous drug. It is insidious." He likewise asserted that the rush to blame aspirin would "prevent the proper study that should be done." He took up the earlier witnesses' descriptions of the differences between causal relationships and correlations and attacked their decision to proceed on the basis of a weak correlation between aspirin and Reye's syndrome: "[T]here is also an association between Reye's syndrome and attending school and there is an association between Reye's syndrome and being Caucasian. You have not seen any recommendations to change either one of those."

Honest Opposition or Inappropriate Influence?

With most of the available evidence coming only from the hearing's transcripts, it is difficult to understand fully Scheuer's and Shacknai's obvious interest in preventing the HHS from warning parents about the possible association between aspirin and Reye's syndrome. The hearing was obviously designed from the start to lambaste the HHS's decision and to reinforce the reputation of aspirin as safe and effective. There appeared to be very little involvement from the other subcommittee members. Other than Scheuer's, the only voice from a member of the House of Representatives to appear in the transcript is Schneider's, and her contributions to the hearing were trivial and at one point entirely off topic.

Scheuer's decision to call the hearings on Reye's syndrome and aspirin are especially odd in light of the commonly offered claim that early 1980s resistance to the adoption of warning labels on aspirin bottles was led by the aspirin manufacturers. Scheuer was, in the words of his former staff director, "an unreconstructed liberal" who had been an outspoken critic of the Vietnam War and had long opposed government interference in private medical issues like abortion and contraception. He had played an important role in the 1980s preserving the Environmental Protection Agency's regulatory powers and in developing Head Start for early education. Especially notable in light of claims that he might have favored industry over public safety was the fact that as chairman of the House Subcommittee on Consumer Protection and Finance he had fought to require seatbelts and airbags against fierce resistance from automakers. At the time of the hearings, he was about halfway through what would ultimately be thirteen terms representing districts in and around New York City.

According to Scheuer's opening statement on the first day of the hearing, his decision to call the hearing was instigated by calls from front-line physicians, not from representatives of the pharmaceutical industry. The Department of Health and Human Services' public announcement of an association between RS and aspirin had provoked physicians around the country to begin contacting him "by the hundreds," with phone calls and letters asking that his subcommittee conduct an investigation. The physicians, he said, "almost unanimously" claimed that the warning was premature and that too little attention had been paid "to the available scientific facts and to the quality of scientific investigations." These claims, Scheuer explained, "had been raised so widely from so many scientific quarters," that nothing short of a full inquiry was appropriate. In this light, Scheuer's concerns about adequate and accurate warning labels on over-the-counter drugs should have aligned nicely with his advocacy of automotive safety and his concern to preserve citizens' ability to make well-informed medical decisions. Those claims, however, stand in stark contrast to his own statement that he was not concerned with preserving physicians' authority but rather with protecting aspirin from being unfairly stigmatized.

Shacknai's intent, on the other hand, appears to be less of a mystery because there is strong circumstantial evidence that he was cultivating an alliance with the pharmaceutical industry that would serve him well when he left public service. At the end of the first day of testimony, Scheuer had made clear just how much influence Shacknai had exerted on the proceedings. "Let me add one word of thanks to our majority counsel, Jonas Shacknai," he said, "who has designed and prepared this hearing with such outstanding professionalism and with such meticulous concern. Thank you."

Shacknai was obviously central to the design and preparation for the two-day hearing on the alleged connection between Reye's syndrome and aspirin, and he played a peculiar role in the story about Reye's syndrome. He had served as the chief aide to the Democrats on the House Subcommittee on Natural Resources, Agriculture Research, and the Environment from 1977 until very shortly after the Reye's syndrome hearing ended. During his service to the House, he had drafted legislation on health care, environmental protection, science policy, and consumer protection. He left House service late in 1982 to become a senior partner in the law firm of Royer, Shacknai, and Mehle, where he represented "over 30 multinational pharmaceutical and medical device concerns, as well as four major industry trade associations." Shacknai also worked "in an executive capacity" for Key Pharmaceuticals, which was acquired in 1986 by Schering-Plough, the pharmaceutical company that had sued to compel the release of the raw data from the Ohio study. In 1988, six years after the hearings on the alleged association between Reye's syndrome and aspirin, he formed Medicis Pharmaceutical Corporation and served as its chairman and chief executive officer for the next twenty-five years. Throughout the 1990s and the first decade of the twenty-first century, he received a number of humanitarian and business awards and was named to two federal cabinet-appointed positions, an NIH advisory council, and the U.S.–Israel Science and Technology Commission. In 2011, Shacknai gained national notoriety when his six-year-old son died from a fatal fall down the staircase of his Colorado mansion. Two days later, Shacknai's girlfriend, Rebecca Mawii Zahau, was found dead at the mansion from what was eventually ruled a suicide. Both deaths aroused suspicions from members of the media, and a second autopsy of Zahau's body was performed that was paid for by the *Dr. Phil Show*. Ultimately, the ugly affair exhibited both Shacknai's complicated personal life and the tremendous wealth he had accumulated.

None of the more recent narratives about the efforts of the aspirin manufacturers to quell concerns about possible links between Reye's syndrome and aspirin take notice of Shacknai or his work with pharmaceutical companies. Standing as he was on the verge of a lucrative career in the pharmaceutical industry, circumstantial evidence suggests that his involvement might have been motivated by something other than a genuine appreciation for the health benefits of aspirin. Both his public efforts and his work behind the scenes significantly shaped the political debates over Reye's syndrome and aspirin. In the fall of 1982, only a few days before Shacknai left public service to advocate for many of the manufacturers of aspirin, there was a stunning shift in the federal government's position on the alleged relationship between aspirin and Reye's syndrome.

CHAPTER SEVEN

The Rise of Labels and the Fall of Reye's

DESPITE A SUMMER-LONG CAMPAIGN in 1982 to discredit the aspirin hypothesis and a carefully organized congressional hearing to showcase claims by the aspirin industry's advocates, federal regulatory agencies continued their plans to require the labeling of aspirin bottles with warnings about Reye's syndrome that fall. On November 20, 1982, the Food and Drug Administration announced plans to require all nonprescription drugs that contained salicylates to carry a warning: "Do not use in persons under 16 years of age with flu or chicken pox unless directed by your doctor." At the same time, the Department of Health and Human Services announced plans to sponsor radio announcements about the possible link between aspirin and RS in an effort to dissuade parents from giving aspirin to ill children.

However, just as the HHS and FDA attempted to move forward with their plans, a growing movement in the United States to limit the regulatory powers of federal agencies halted them. In the early 1980s, just as the first evidence of a relationship between aspirin and RS was published, a powerful deregulation movement emerged in Washington. Throughout most of Ronald Reagan's presidency, government agencies were increasingly denied the ability to regulate in favor of the consumer, the environment, or the public's health. As the National Consumer League complained in 1983, "Almost every area of vital concern to consumers was adversely affected by the Administration's relentless drive to deny the role of government in protecting citizens." The deregulation movement provided an important backdrop to the story of Reye's syndrome and the efforts by advocates of the aspirin hypothesis to encourage the government to mandate warning labels on aspirin bottles.

Perhaps even more influential than the efforts of the Aspirin Foundation or the Committee for the Care of Children in slowing the effort to label aspirin bottles was the much quieter work done by advocates for deregulation like Jim Tozzi, a former official in the Office of Management and Budget (OMB). Tozzi has long been a powerful Washington insider, and lately he has received a great deal of attention from authors who lament what they perceive as an inappropriate politicization of science. For example, William Kleinknecht, author of *The Man Who Sold the World: Ronald Reagan and the Betrayal of Main Street America*, called Tozzi "the kind of person even his political enemies find hard not to like" before branding him "a one-man fifth column embedded in the bureaucracy." Similarly, Chris Mooney, author of *The Republican War on Science*, described in detail how Tozzi "has managed to change the very rules of the regulatory game itself." While Tozzi claims his overarching goal is merely to "regulate the regulators, preventing agencies from arbitrarily releasing or relying on bad information," Mooney reported that many of his critics consider his strategy an attempt to create "paralysis by analysis." That was certainly the case with Reye's syndrome, as Tozzi played a critical role in slowing the effort to mandate labels on aspirin bottles to warn of the drug's possible connection to Reye's syndrome.

Tozzi had come to Washington in 1964 with a Ph.D. in economics and business administration to work at the Department of Defense. Eight years later he moved to the OMB, a powerful cabinet-level office in the executive branch. The OMB's main function is to assist in the preparation of annual federal budgets, but its real power comes in its charge to measure and assess the quality of various federal agencies' programs, policies, and procedures. In this role, it has the capacity to dictate the actual functioning of the federal government. As chief of the environmental branch of the OMB in the Nixon and Ford administrations, Tozzi was considered "the single most influential person in the U.S. in shaping environmental policy nationally." Throughout the late 1970s, as the executive branch swung from Republican to Democratic and back to Republican presidents, Tozzi's influence as a reformer of regulatory agencies grew. An early advocate of market-based approaches to government reform, he criticized administrators in the Environmental Protection Agency who he believed too frequently adopted costly, ineffective regulations. Most authorities on the subject say that Tozzi was critical in the passage of the powerful 1980 Paperwork Reduction Act and the associated creation of the OMB Office of Information and Regulatory Affairs (OIRA). In a 1981 interview, Tozzi said that he had "cashed in every chit" he had to pass the Paperwork Reduction Act; for his efforts, he was named the first director of the OIRA.

Known to his staff as "the Ayatollah" for his intense demands on them and by some of his enemies as "Stealth" for his ability to reach "his target, while shielding his whereabouts from adversaries," Tozzi has long been a powerful force in Washington. In the early 1980s, in the midst of the political debates over labeling aspirin bottles with warnings about Reye's syndrome, Tozzi made the leap from seasoned bureaucrat to private consultant. In the spring of 1983, he founded a new consulting firm, Multinational Business Service Corp., and became a consultant to the law firm of Beveridge and Diamond. Three years later, he cofounded Federal Focus, a nonprofit organization supported by the tobacco company Philip Morris, which has served as the funding source for dozens of new nonprofit policy institutes. These organizations, with names like the Center for Epidemiological Studies and the Center for Regulatory Effectiveness, have shaped the ways in which the federal government weighs questions of risk, especially as they relate to public health issues, by funneling money from Philip Morris through the innocuous-sounding Federal Focus.

On the eve of his departure from public service, Tozzi stalled the effort to label aspirin bottles with warnings about Reye's syndrome. At some point in 1982, Joseph White had learned of the OMB's power to prevent the FDA from mandating labels, so five representatives from the Aspirin Foundation met with Tozzi after working hours at the OMB headquarters. They presented Tozzi with the name of a physician—whose name I have not been able to determine—who opposed labeling. Tozzi later told a reporter that this physician's views "greatly influenced him." While almost everyone else in the OMB associated with the question of labeling believed it was a prudent public health action, Tozzi began working to undermine the plan. He eschewed traditional methods of issuing memos, making public pronouncements, or offering congressional testimony, instead preferring phone calls and private meetings. As Tozzi said with a grin in an interview with the *Washington Post* in 1981, "I don't want to leave fingerprints." After talking to the unnamed physician, he called officials at the FDA to tell them, "You have not made your case."

For a public statement on the matter, Tozzi turned to Jonah Shacknai, the architect of the September 1982 congressional hearings that attacked the aspirin hypothesis and its supporters. Less than three weeks after the hearing, Shacknai published a polemic piece in the *Wall Street Journal.* He attacked HHS secretary Schweiker for announcing plans to require warning labels on aspirin-containing products and to begin a public service campaign. He called the four studies on the relationship between aspirin and Reye's syndrome "significantly flawed" and biased. "Many doctors with firsthand experience with Reye's, as well as the Reye's Syndrome Association," Shacknai claimed, "have opposed the HHS effort because they believe that parents and physicians will treat Reye's as a preventable illness and, consequently, will be less alert to its symptoms." There is little evidence to support these bold claims, unless one mistakenly accepts that the carefully selected pool of witnesses from the previous month's trial were actually representative of the medical community. Within a week of the article's publication, Shacknai had resigned as majority counsel and began working for eleven pharmaceutical companies and the American Reye's Syndrome Association, the industry-funded RS advocacy group.

Armed with Shacknai's op-ed piece and the Aspirin Foundation's report from its RS Working Group that had been published in *Pediatrics,* Tozzi wrote a memorandum to Christopher DeMuth, Reagan's so-called deregulation czar and Tozzi's superior at OMB. DeMuth later explained that Schackai's article and his reading of the testimony in the hearing that Shacknai had orchestrated were in line with opinions he heard from his wife, who was a pediatrician. Early in November 1982, DeMuth called HHS secretary Schweiker and urged him to reconsider the order to begin labeling aspirin bottles with warnings about Reye's syndrome. He told

Schweiker that if HHS would not withdraw plans to require labels, the OMB would effectively veto the HHS's order by declaring that its costs outweighed its potential benefits.

As representatives from the aspirin industry encouraged regulators to abandon plans for labeling, they also pressured leaders of the American Academy of Pediatrics to reverse their organization's stance. After already having heard threats of a lawsuit from the Schering-Plough representatives when they first called for RS warning labels on aspirin bottles early in 1982, leaders of the AAP were again threatened that fall. On November 8, 1982, the AAP's executive board held a hastily arranged telephone conference and reversed its position on the issue of labeling. Two members of the organizations' Infectious Disease Committee—Edward Mortimer, Jr., and Vincent Fulginiti—resigned in protest. Mortimer, who had been the lead author on a 1962 paper connecting aspirin with the symptoms that would later be associated with Reye's syndrome, said that the reversal came in response to "heavy pressure from certain members of the academy who were recruited by the aspirin industry." Elsewhere, Mortimer said that he was "distressed" that the board had "pulled the rug out from underneath so many people who have studied this issue so carefully. . . . I believe that their statement very sadly is a consequence of rather considerable direct and indirect pressure from aspirin manufacturers."

Given the AAP's apparent reversal and threats of veto from the OMB, on November 18, 1982, Schweiker announced that he was withdrawing plans to require that aspirin manufacturers label their products with warnings about possible links to Reye's syndrome. He was silent about the pressure he received from the OMB and asserted that the basis for his decision was instead the AAP's recent statement. "This," he said, "is the first time concerns have been raised by an independent scientific body, and it is critical that they be resolved." Reflecting Schweiker's assertions that his agency's inaction was the result of a lack of scientific consensus, the *New York Times* concluded its story about the reversal by stating, "There is a dispute in the scientific community over whether or not evidence is strong enough to prove a link between aspirin and the disease." Similarly, the *Washington Post* reported that there was a "'scientific dispute' over the dangers of aspirin use in children with chicken pox or flu." Given the earlier statements from the CDC—the government agency charged with studying such issues—these characterizations were, at best, overstatements of a relatively small number of lingering questions about the relationship between aspirin and Reye's syndrome or shortcomings with the existing studies.

Nonetheless, Schweiker announced that more research was necessary before the HHS could make any recommendations. He ordered the U.S. Public Health Service to make recommendations to him about how to conduct this research. The result was a pilot study followed by a main study that attempted to more clearly demonstrate what the four state studies had already shown: that aspirin use by children with viral illnesses was strongly correlated with the emergence of the symptoms associated with Reye's syndrome. As well designed as these studies were to be, however, they were increasingly difficult to conduct because the incidence of Reye's syndrome was rapidly declining. For his part, Joseph White of the Aspirin Foundation said that he was happy to see that the government was "going to go forward on a somewhat more reasonable basis and look to the design of a proper study."

In the end, aspirin industry representatives exercised considerable influence in the HHS's decisions to halt plans to require warning labels on aspirin bottles. Jim Tozzi wielded enough influence to launch him out of public service and into a lucrative new career as a private consultant, where he continued to undersell the tremendous power he wielded inside the beltway. A year later, in an obvious attempt to camouflage his role in the events that led to Schweiker's reversal, Tozzi told a reporter, "Without OMB's involvement, the rule would have gone out. Everybody knew it would never get past those mongrels at OMB."

Public Citizen and the Aspirin Hypothesis

The advocates of deregulation had not gone unopposed. A popular movement to use government regulation to protect consumers from abuse in the marketplace had long worked to empower federal agencies, and the issue of labeling aspirin became a battleground for consumer advocates and proponents of deregulation. With some acknowledged level of uncertainty about a causal relationship between aspirin and Reye's syndrome and a rising tide of deregulation in Washington, advocates of the aspirin hypothesis portrayed themselves as struggling to protect children from the deadly and mysterious ailment. Beginning in the months that followed the first assertive statements from the AAP and the HHS about the identified relationship between aspirin and Reye's syndrome in the spring of 1982, consumer advocates took up the effort to force aspirin manufacturers to label their products with warnings about Reye's syndrome.

The consumer movement in the United States had begun shortly after the turn of the twentieth century, casting itself as the protector of the average American consumer against the tyranny and abuse of business interests. Originally linked with progressivism and driven by a new generation of investigative journalists, the first wave of the consumer movement was typified by Upton Sinclair's *The Jungle* and the passage of the Pure Food and Drug Act of 1906. By the 1930s, the movement had shifted to focus on attacking false claims in advertising, and the 1938 Wheeler-Lea Act empowered the Federal Trade Commission to prohibit unfair or deceptive acts or practices and unfair methods of competition. The acts of 1906 and 1938 together provided reformers and activists with a legal basis to pursue lawsuits against companies that made false claims or harmful products. The modern consumer movement, however, did not emerge until the social movements of the 1960s and 1970s provided a broad base of activists and reform-minded consumers who looked to the government for enhanced protection from harmful products.

Throughout the first half of the 1980s, the fight in Washington to force the government to warn parents about a potential relationship between aspirin and Reye's syndrome was led by the nonprofit consumer-rights group Public Citizen. The organization had been formed in 1971 by Ralph Nader to provide a voice for the American citizen in Washington. It has long sought corporate accountability through robust government regulations, particularly in the areas of health care, transportation, and nuclear energy. Public Citizen's slogan is "Corporations have their lobbyists in Washington DC. The People need advocates too." The organization continues its work today, focusing primarily on public interest lawsuits.

Public Citizen's efforts to force the government to require that aspirin bottles be labeled to warn of Reye's syndrome was spearheaded by Sidney Wolfe, who cofounded and directed Public Citizen's Health Research Group (HRG). Wolfe was a physician who had worked at the National Institutes of Health on research on blood clotting and alcoholism. He met Nader at a professional meeting in the late 1960s and began serving as an advisor to him on health issues. When Nader formed Public Citizen in 1971, he asked Wolfe to set up the HRG, which was intended to "improve the public health by using research-based advocacy." He directed the HRG for more than three decades before stepping down in 2013. In a public statement about Wolfe's retirement, Robert Weissman, president of Public Citizen, said, "Sid Wolfe has never backed down in the face of enormous industry and government pressure, and the result is that our country is safer and healthier."

Frustrated by the FDA's slow pace to label aspirin bottles in light of what Wolfe and his colleagues considered an overwhelming amount of scientific evidence pointing to a relationship between aspirin and Reye's syndrome, the HRG and the American Public Health Association filed suit on May 17, 1982 in the District of Columbia's federal district court. The suit sought a court order to force the FDA to require manufacturers to begin immediately labeling aspirin bottles with a warning about Reye's syndrome. The circuit court of appeals heard the case in December 1983 and issued its ruling six months later. The court reported that, although the "exact cause of Reye's syndrome is unknown," many people in the medical community had suspected for at least twenty years that the cause might be aspirin. It was true that twenty years earlier Mortimer and Lepow had suggested a relationship between salicylates and the symptoms that would later be associated with RS, but the court's assessment was too generous. Remember that throughout the 1970s the index of suspicion for aspirin was so low for aspirin that Starko and her colleagues had a difficult time publishing both their initial findings and their later pathology discoveries.

After recounting the studies from Arizona, Michigan, and Ohio in the early 1980s, the court described the CDC's early actions to encourage parents and medical providers to avoid aspirin use whenever possible with children who had chicken pox or influenza. Subsequent FDA actions reinforced the CDC's warning, and it appeared that government officials had been slowly moving toward the requirement that aspirin be labeled to warn about its apparent association with Reye's syndrome by issuing an advance notice of the proposal. In the midst of this, the court reported, the HRG claimed that the "FDA's decision to promulgate an advanced notice of proposed rulemaking instead of issuing a rule requiring a Reye's syndrome warning label for products containing aspirin" constituted an unreasonable delay in carrying out the plan to label aspirin bottles that was announced in the fall of 1982.

The court approached the HRG's request with great trepidation. As a rule, courts are not inclined to involve themselves in the day-to-day functions of government agencies or in the regulatory process in general. So, the court asserted that the HRG's plea "demands a great deal of the court," in requesting that it "decide itself that aspirin products without a Reye's syndrome warning label are misbranded" or that the HHS and FDA were not adequately and immediately fulfilling their promise to require that aspirin bottles be labeled. Even given its general hesitation about involving itself in agency business, the court said, "The facts do evoke some sympathy for [the] HRG's claim." There did seem to be considerable evidence that aspirin was causally involved in Reye's syndrome, and both the FDA and the HHS "appear to continue to view the evidence linking salicylates and Reye's syndrome as sufficiently strong to justify an education campaign alerting physicians and parents to the danger." The court could in fact hurry along the process of producing new regulations in certain circumstances. "Quite simply," the court quoted from a 1975 case brought by Ralph Nader against the FCC, "excessive delay saps the public confidence in an agency's ability to discharge its responsibilities . . ." Similarly, quoting the decision rendered in another case brought by the HRG, the court asserted, "Delays that might be altogether reasonable in the sphere of economic regulation are less tolerable when human lives are at stake."

HRG's request to the appeals court engaged a set of judicial principles that had developed throughout the late 1960s and early 1970s concerning courts' capacities to review or coerce agency action. Two of the tools relevant to judicial oversight of agency actions were particularly relevant to the HRG's request: finality and ripeness. Both conditions must be fulfilled in order for the court to review an agency's decision or compel an agency to take action. "Finality" refers to a situation in which there are no "additional steps or procedures necessary before enforcement or implementation can be undertaken." "Ripeness" is met when the court decides that the issues at hand are ready to be resolved by a judicial decision and the plaintiff can demonstrate that a hardship will be suffered if the court does not review the case. For the court to be able to render a decision in favor of the HRG's petition, it would have to first decide that the requirements of both finality and ripeness had been met. Lacking that determination, the court would decline to issue a decision about the pace toward requiring labeling that the FDA appeared to be making.

Despite recognizing that "the law does provide means by which the interests of regulatory beneficiaries can be protected from the adverse effects of delays in agency action," the appeals court concluded that it could not render a decision in favor of the HRG's request because the case failed to meet either the finality or the ripeness requirements for the court to review agency actions. It failed the finality test because the FDA's statements in the spring and summer of 1982 were superseded later that year when the agency announced that it was "'considering proposing' a rule requiring aspirin warning labels and was proceeding by way of an advance notice." The FDA's statements earlier that year were therefore judged to be "facially preparatory" because "supervening events have overtaken" the earlier statements about the agency's intentions to require warning labels. The appeals court thus reaffirmed the district court's refusal to address the question of whether or not aspirin bottles should be labeled to warn about potential links between aspirin and Reye's syndrome.

Although the court refused to overturn the lower court's decision, it did find serious questions "with respect to whether FDA is resolving within 'a reasonable time' the issues the HRG has raised." Based on the evidence presented by the HRG, the appeals court concluded, "The current record strongly suggests that the pace of agency decision-making is unreasonably dilatory. All scientific evidence in the record points to a link between salicylates and Reye's syndrome, and the agency has itself credited this evidence at least to the extent of conducting an education campaign to warn physicians and parents of the potential risks that salicylates pose." The court stated that these conclusions were "particularly troubling" because "the pace of agency decision-making may jeopardize the lives of children" and the appeals court remanded the case to the district court to determine if the process has been "unreasonably delayed." If the district court found that the FDA had been moving too slowly, it could "fashion an appropriate remedy" that could include an order to begin immediately and proceed expeditiously or require periodic reports to the court.

Studying Reye's Syndrome As It Disappears

While regulators and politicians continued to debate the merits of claims about the association between Reye's syndrome and aspirin, researchers and public health officials undertook first a pilot and then a full study that they hoped would overcome all the criticisms launched against the Arizona, Ohio, and Michigan studies. Reye's syndrome cases typically occur between December and April, so by the time HHS Secretary Schweiker made his announcement in mid-November 1982 that more studies were needed, it was too late to organize a study for the 1983 season. But by the next fall, a coalition of over a dozen researchers organized into the Public Health Service Reye Syndrome Task Force had a plan in place to study the relationship between Reye's syndrome and ten different categories of medications, including salicylates. They published the results of their pilot study in the fall of 1985 and the report of their main study in the spring of 1987. Both supported the conclusions from the four earlier state studies. Children with viral illnesses who consumed aspirin were much more likely to develop Reye's syndrome than were non-aspirin–consuming children with viral illnesses.

The report from the pilot phase began with a blunt admission: "As with many epidemiologic studies, concerns have been expressed regarding methodologic issues and the limitation of these four case studies . . ."

These concerns included some of the most pointed criticisms that had emerged from the Aspirin Foundation and in Scheuer's 1982 house subcommittee hearings. Among them were allegations that parents did not accurately recall the medications they administered to their sick children, that the control group had not suffered from similar antecedent illnesses as had the children who had developed RS, and that at least some of the reported cases of Reye's syndrome had been misclassified.

Both the pilot and the main studies were every bit as rigorous as the researchers were capable of making them. They established strict criteria for eligibility of suspected cases of Reye's syndrome, and the controls were carefully chosen on the basis of location and demographic data. Instead of gathering information about prodromal illnesses from parents generally, the researchers drew from in-depth interviews with the people who had cared for the children. Professional interviewers, employed and trained by an independent contractor, conducted all interviews, and they established careful timelines for the children's illnesses and for their consumption of medications throughout their illnesses. Drawing representative researchers from the CDC, the FDA, the NIH, and the HHS, the two studies were designed and overseen by some of the most experienced investigators of Reye's syndrome, including Eugene Hurwitz, who had run the Ohio study, and Lawrence Schonberger at the CDC, who had helped guide much of the work done in the four state studies.

The pilot study, the report of which was published in the *New England Journal of Medicine* in the fall of 1985, collected information from sixteen pediatric health-care centers in eleven states. The researchers identified thirty cases of Reye's syndrome and 145 control subjects divided into four different kinds of control groups. They found ten different medications, including acetaminophen, various cold and flu relievers like guaifenesin or pseudoephedrine hydrochloride, and salicylates, that were consumed by at least 20 percent of the study subjects. Almost all (93 percent) of the children who had eventually developed Reye's syndrome had taken aspirin, while the average for the four control groups was less than 50 percent (Table 1). The researchers concluded that there was "a strong association between Reye's syndrome

	Children Who Contracted RS N = 30	Controls N = 145
Acetaminophen	27%	67%
Alcohol	50%	54%
Camphor	10%	13%
Chlorpheniramine maleate	20%	23%
Dextromethorphan hydrobromide	23%	36%
Guaifenesin	23%	26%
Phenylephrine hydrochloride	20%	13%
Phenylpropanolamine hydrochloride	40%	34%
Pseudoephedrine hydrochloride	20%	18%
Salicylates	93%	46%

Table 1. Generic Components of Medications Administered to 20% or More of the Children During Prodromal Illness (Pilot Study)

and the use of salicylates during the antecedent illness of Reye's syndrome, consistent with the results reported in earlier studies." The pilot report closed by reporting that a larger study that involved more that fifty pediatric care centers was currently under way.

The main study appeared eighteen months later in the *Journal of the American Medical Association*, and it demonstrated an even stronger relationship between aspirin and Reye's syndrome. While on average only about 38 percent of the controls had received aspirin during their prodromal illness, more than 96 percent of the children who eventually contracted RS had been given aspirin. (Table 2) The conclusion was that the odds of a child with a viral illness developing Reye's syndrome was far, far greater if that child had received aspirin. The main study concluded, "Thus, this study reinforces the importance of reducing the use of aspirin (and possibly all salicylates) for the treatment of children with chickenpox and influenza-like illness to further reduce the incidence of Reye's syndrome in the United States."

Conspicuous among the data presented in the both the pilot and the

	Children Who Contracted RS N = 27	Controls N = 140
Acetaminophen	30%	88%
Alcohol	44%	56%
Amoxicillin	7%	9%
Caffeine	22%	7%
Camphor	15%	14%
Chlorpheniramine maleate	22%	26%
Dextromethorphan hydrobromide	30%	41%
Eucalyptus oil	30%	23%
Guaifenesin	22%	36%
Menthol	41%	31%
Phenol	11%	14%
Phenylephrine hydrochloride	15%	18%
Phenylpropanolamine hydrochloride	19%	39%
Pseudoephedrine hydrochloride	30%	32%
Salicylates	96%	38%

TABLE 2. Generic Components of Medications Administered to 20% or More of the Children During Prodromal Illness (Main Study)

main studies were the rapidly dwindling numbers of children diagnosed with Reye's syndrome each year (see the graph on page 160). Reported cases had peaked in 1980 with 555, but fell away quickly throughout the 1980s. The increasing rarity of the ailment—even as the researchers welcomed it—represented a significant challenge to their efforts to document and explore the relationship between aspirin and RS. The researchers who had conducted the Ohio study during the 1979 and 1980 seasons had identified 154 cases in just one state, and the two Michigan studies included fifty-six and twelve cases. However, even with all of the federal and state resources available for the pilot study conducted by the U.S. Public Health Service during the 1984 season, researchers were only able to identify thirty cases across eleven states. The main study, which

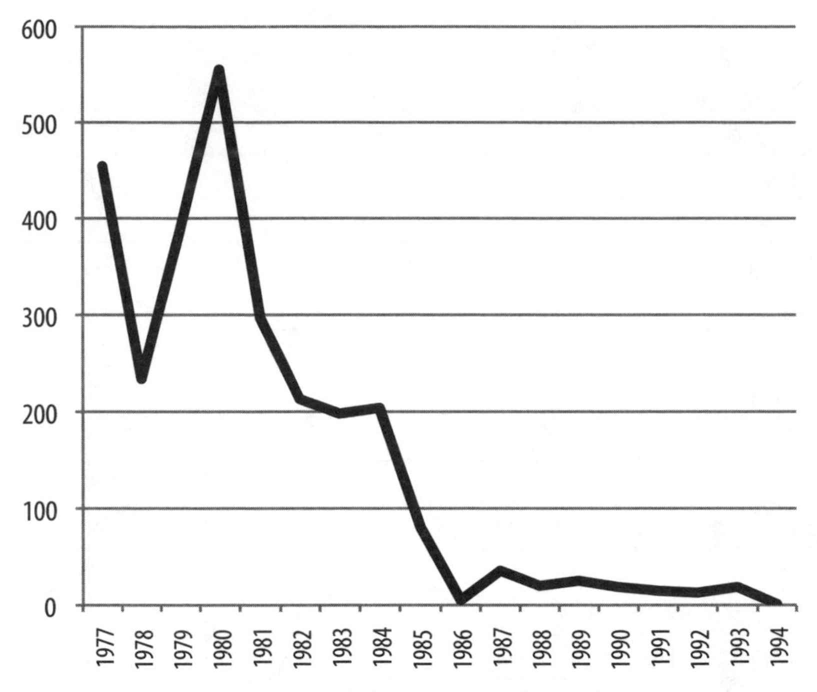

Annual Number of Reported Cases of Reye's Syndrome, 1977–1994

covered two full seasons and fifteen states, included even fewer cases: researchers identified only twenty-seven.

There also emerged evidence that showed that the incidence of Reye's syndrome was falling in concert with the decreasing use of aspirin in children and, despite the stalled labeling mandate, there was a growing awareness among parents that aspirin might cause the disorder. Even without warning labels on aspirin bottles, parents had learned about a possible link between aspirin and Reye's syndrome through a series of state and federal educational campaigns and an aggressive effort by the AAP to encourage pediatricians to educate parents about the relationship. Early in 1986, as the Public Health Service Reye Syndrome Task Force was compiling data for its final report, several of the researchers who had produced the Michigan study published results of a study on aspirin use. Interviews with 210 mothers (and one father) over a two-year period about their families' medication use and their knowledge of Reye's syndrome showed a substantial decline in aspirin consumption by children. Between 1981 and 1983 the percentage of parents who gave their children aspirin fell from 56 percent to 25 percent. Younger parents, they found, gave aspirin less often, and more than half of the parents who were aware of the association between aspirin and Reye's syndrome reported that they stopped using aspirin because of concerns about RS. These findings were corroborated by a second study published a year later that drew from pharmaceutical marketing research data to show likewise that there were sharp decreases in the purchase and use of children's aspirin throughout the early 1980s.

The final report of the U.S. Public Health Service's study was accompanied by an editorial by Edward A. Mortimer, Jr., who had quit the AAP's Infectious Disease Committee in disgust in 1982 when the organization waffled on its earlier statement about the association between aspirin and Reye's syndrome. Mortimer wrote that between the time when the first, tentative warnings about Reye's syndrome and aspirin appeared in 1980 and the main study's final report was published in 1987, 1,003 cases of Reye's syndrome were reported to the CDC. Of those, 291 of the children had died, and it was likely that more than two hundred of the survivors had suffered permanent brain damage. Later authors would increase the number of cases during the five years that the federal government waited to begin labeling aspirin bottles to over five thousand and the deaths from RS to 1,470. They arrived at these figures by multiplying the reported numbers by five on the basis of a statement by the head of the Division of Viral and Infectious Diseases at the CDC, Ali Khan, who had estimated that only "about 20% of all cases are recorded under its surveillance system," and that 33 percent to 40 percent of the unreported cases were fatal. Mortimer's editorial marked a fundamental shift in the discussion about Reye's syndrome and aspirin, as researchers and public health officials went on the offensive against what they viewed as abusive industry representatives, sluggish bureaucrats, and politicians who chose to protect bottom lines instead of children. Over the next two decades, the modern narrative about "paralysis by analysis" and junk science emerged, and the story of Reye's syndrome become a centerpiece of the narrative about the politicization of science in the United States.

CHAPTER EIGHT

Labels, At Last

IN JANUARY 1985, A MONTH after the results of the U.S. Public Health Service's pilot study were published, the Public Citizen's Health Research Group again petitioned the FDA to require warning labels, and the new HHS secretary, Margaret Heckler, sidestepped OMB oversight by asking aspirin manufacturers to voluntarily place warning labels on their products. At the same time, she expanded the HHS's public education campaign, which was met by little animosity from either deregulators or the aspirin industry. She also asked that manufacturers remove from their labels any suggestion that aspirin should be used to treat flu or chicken pox in children or teenagers. Schering-Plough and Bayer quickly announced that they would cooperate with the voluntary labeling program, but both continued to assert that they were unconvinced that there was sufficient evidence to show any relationship—much less a causal one—between aspirin and Reye's syndrome. In an obvious attempt to demonstrate cooperation while continuing to ignore the results of five different studies that demonstrated a relationship between aspirin and Reye's syndrome, Joseph White of the Aspirin Foundation said, "We agreed we would go forward with our part of it without waiting for the data to be made available." By the end of the month, every major aspirin manufacturer had pledged support for voluntary labeling that would warn parents not to give aspirin to children but would not mention aspirin's possible link to Reye's syndrome.

By the mid-1980s, American industries and the U.S. government had established a routine way for industry to police itself that enabled the federal government to avoid having to enact and enforce regulations.

Examples of self-regulation stretch as far back as medieval times, when guilds policed the markets, measures, and quality of their members' products. Modern self-regulation emerged in the early twentieth century among advertisers who recognized the potential damage that unrestrained false advertising would have on the public's willingness to trust advertisers' claims. By the 1930s, following the publications of books like Stuart Chase and F. J. Schlink's *Your Money's Worth* and Arthur Kallet and F. J. Schlink's *100,000,000 Guinea Pigs* as well as growing calls for governmental regulation of advertising, the Copeland Bill threatened to increase federal regulation of advertising by shifting the responsibility for regulation from the Federal Trade Commission to the Food and Drug Administration, which would have been empowered to enact strict regulations. To prevent this, the aspirin industry vocally adopted measures to regulate itself.

In the 1960s, when Reye's syndrome was first described, public discontent over corporate abuses was high, and many industries responded by recommitting themselves to self-regulation in order to avoid formal regulation by the federal government. Nowhere was the use of self-regulation more evident than in the movie industry. In 1922, the U.S. film industry had adopted the Motion Picture Production Code, popularly known as the Hays Code after Will H. Hays, who had the unique qualifications of being the chairman of the Republican National Committee, a Presbyterian deacon, the U.S. postmaster, and the head of the Motion Picture Producers and Distributors of America. The code was an explicit effort to respond to growing calls for censorship of the motion picture industry and to prevent the passage of state or federal laws that would have regulated the content of films. In the 1960s, the Hays Code was abandoned under increasingly intense pressure from filmmakers and the public, both of whom viewed it as unreasonably prudish. A new industry-wide rating system went into effect at the end of 1968 that rated a film G, for general audiences; M, for mature audiences; R, for restricted to those over seventeen; or X, for sexually explicit. Over the next forty years the ratings system evolved slightly but today it still maintains its original structure and, more important, its original intent to allow the movie industry to regulate itself and stave off state or federal oversight.

Throughout the twentieth century, a number of other U.S. industries have turned to self-regulation when they were threatened by the possibility of government regulation or by critical public opinion. Most notable among these were the food, tobacco, forestry, fisheries, and firearm industries, but occasional bouts of concern over public welfare have continued to threaten the independence of self-regulated industries. On the other hand, periods of focused deregulation—like the one that dominated Ronald Reagan's presidency—saw increased reliance on self-regulation. Perhaps the best example from the 1980s was the work of the Parents Music Resource Center (PMRC).

The PMRC was formed in 1985 by Tipper Gore (wife of Al Gore, then senator and later vice president), Susan Baker (wife of treasury secretary James Baker), Sally Nevius (wife of the former Washington city council chairman John Nevius), and Pam Howar (wife of a prominent DC realtor). Known as the Washington Wives, the group led an effort to coerce the U.S. music industry to adopt guidelines similar to the film rating system in order to prevent children from hearing objectionable lyrics in popular music. They identified the "Filthy Fifteen," a list of songs that they deemed objectionable because they contained sex, drug, violent, or occult references, and their work encouraged the removal of some albums and magazines from a few department store chains. In September 1985, after publishing articles in the *Washington Post* and *Newsweek*, the PMRC members' concerns were examined in a Senate hearing before the Committee on Commerce, Science and Transportation, of which Al Gore was a member (as was Bob Packwood, who would later resign from the Senate under threat of expulsion after allegations of sexual harassment, abuse, and assault emerged). Opposing witnesses included Frank Zappa, John Denver, and Dee Snider (the lead singer from the heavy metal band Twisted Sister), all of whom gave strikingly persuasive testimony against labeling. Nonetheless, only a month later, the Recording Industry Association of America announced that it would begin labeling albums that contained material that some Americans might find objectionable.

The adoption of self-enforced regulations forestalls or prevents the enactment of government regulations and calms public pressures, but only if the industries make a reasonable effort at crafting and enforcing guidelines to protect the public welfare. When industry's actions and public health objectives do not coincide, industry groups are incentivized to promise change, but to create weak standards, enforce them laxly, and slow their adoption whenever possible. Many critics of the compromise offered by HHS Secretary Heckler believed that whatever good might come from the voluntary labeling program would be undermined by the aspirin industry's decision to add a label that only weakly alluded to the suspected link between aspirin and Reye's syndrome. In the midst of the Reagan-era deregulation movement, just as the Washington Wives were seeking to protect American children from the supposedly damaging effects of some popular music, many alleged that the aspirin industry was preventing parents from learning about the possibly deadly effects of giving their children aspirin.

Just as the PMRC members turned to Capitol Hill and asked for a hearing that would bring to light the threat of popular music, Representative Henry Waxman and Senator Howard Metzenbaum introduced a bill proposing the Emergency Reye's Syndrome Prevention Act of 1985 in the House and Senate, which would have forced the Department of Health and Human Services to enact labeling regulations. Waxman and Metzenbaum held a press conference at the end of February 1985 announcing their concern that the voluntary aspirin labeling program "appears [to be] failing," so "stronger steps are needed to protect the public." Only one manufacturer—Schering—had moved quickly enough with their labeling efforts to satisfy Waxman and Metzenbaum. They introduced legislation on February 28, 1985, to force the immediate labeling of aspirin bottles with a warning about Reye's syndrome but recognized that Congress could not move quickly enough to get the labels on bottles during the current flu season. However, Waxman said, "[T]he introduction of legislation requiring harsher warning language could have the effect of speeding industry compliance with the voluntary program." To further encourage voluntary compliance, he explained that he intended to schedule a hearing on the legislation before his House subcommittee. It proved different in almost every way from the House subcommittee meeting that Rep. James Scheuer had chaired less than three years earlier.

Representative Waxman's Hearing on Aspirin & Reye's Syndrome

Henry Waxman, the liberal Democratic Representative from California's 33rd congressional district, was first elected to Congress in 1974 after serving three terms in the California Assembly. Born and reared in California, he had earned a bachelor's degree and a law degree from the University of California at Los Angeles. Throughout the 1980s and 1990s, Waxman led a number of investigations and legislative efforts related to health and the environment, including measures concerning HIV/AIDS, pollution, and health insurance coverage. In 1984 he cosponsored the Hatch-Waxman Act, which encouraged the manufacture of generic drugs and established federal regulation of them. In 2003, Waxman released a report from the Oversight and Government Reform Committee that accused President George W. Bush of politicizing science, making abstinence-based sex education programs appear more effective than they really were. Forty years after he was first elected to Congress, Waxman was one of the most influential members, and he was actively involved in issues related to health and the environment until his retirement from Congress in 2014.

Waxman opened his subcommittee's hearing on aspirin, Reye's syndrome, and warning labels on the morning of March 15, 1985. He stated that the purpose of the hearing was to examine "the adequacy of steps taken by the Department of Health and Human Services and the aspirin industry in the past few months to alert the public to the possible dangers associated with the use of aspirin during certain childhood diseases." Waxman had raised concerns earlier that year that the voluntary labeling program might be insufficient to protect children, and in January 1985 had requested that HHS Secretary Heckler report to his subcommittee about whatever progress had been made in labeling aspirin bottles. In his opening statement before the March hearing, Waxman announced that the "voluntary effort is failing on four counts." First, the labels that the HHS and representatives from aspirin manufacturers had negotiated were inadequate and vague; in fact, they did not even mention Reye's syndrome. Second, there was no necessity that the labels be prominently displayed on aspirin bottles. Third, the industry had been slow to label the bottles, so most of the aspirin sold during the 1985 flu season would not have included the warning label, as insufficient and ineffective as it might be. Fourth, some aspirin manufacturers were not even part of the voluntary agreement and would have continued to sell aspirin in bottles without warning labels. Waxman concluded that in light of the "strong and consistent" evidence of a link between aspirin and Reye's syndrome, which had been further supported by the recently released PHS pilot study and the IOM's review, as well as HHS's apparent unwillingness to require aspirin manufacturers to warn about Reye's syndrome, "Congress must act."

Waxman's short opening statement moved quickly into a dialogue with Metzenbaum, who had introduced similar legislation in the Senate. Metzenbaum emphasized researchers' high level of certainty about a causal relationship between Reye's syndrome and aspirin. "Here we have a situation where we know the problem," he asserted. "It is indisputable. The facts are there." Unlike many other health problems in which we don't know the cause, he stated, "we know that the ingestion of aspirin by children when they have chicken pox or influenza does have the potential to harm the children. That is irrefutable, and we can prevent it, so why not." After insisting that researchers were certain that aspirin caused Reye's syndrome, Metzenbaum turned his attention to the HHS and the voluntary agreement that Heckler negotiated with representatives from some aspirin manufacturers. "We have seen," he concluded, "that voluntary cooperation doesn't work."

Waxman thanked Metzenbaum and made clear their shared agreement about the inadequacy of Heckler's response to the alleged threat aspirin posed to children. "I was astounded," Waxman said, "at this voluntary agreement that the Secretary negotiated." It did not include all aspirin companies, the agreed-upon labels were weak and uninformative, and the labels would not appear until well after the current influenza season. "Voluntary efforts are fine if they work, but voluntary efforts that don't have the chance of really reaching the public are meaningless." They also expressed serious concern about the industry's unwillingness to accept what they described as "overwhelming" evidence of the link between aspirin and RS. Metzenbaum bluntly attacked the aspirin manufacturers: "Why are they using that kind of political maneuvering to do it on a voluntary basis, are we going to affect their sales that much? So what? So what? . . . What bothers me is that here is a known problem, not just a fictitious one, not one that is a figment of the imagination, and if it is a known problem why the hell don't they do something about it and why do we have to use our efforts to pass legislation to force them to do something that they should be doing on their own."

Given the striking difference between Waxman's 1985 hearing on the relationship between aspirin and Reye's syndrome and Scheuer's hearing two and a half years earlier, it is surprising to see Scheuer's name in the transcript of the 1985 hearing. At its start, Waxman recognized Scheuer and offered him an opportunity to make a statement, but Scheuer declined. A few moments later, after Waxman and Metzenbaum had finished describing the possible connection between aspirin and Reye's syndrome as "indisputable," Scheuer graciously thanked Metzenbaum for attending and complimented him as someone who "can always be counted upon not only for wisdom and insight and high order of intellectual acumen, but sheer unadulterated guts, and that is frequently a scarce commodity in these precincts." As the hearing progressed, it quickly became apparent that Scheuer's position on the alleged relationship between aspirin and Reye's syndrome had changed quite radically over the previous two and a half years.

The differences in the organization of the 1982 and 1985 hearings demonstrated the stark differences in Scheuer's and Waxman's original intents in calling the hearings. Scheuer had organized his 1982 subcommittee meeting by calling experts who were critical of the alleged link between aspirin and Reye's syndrome, then grilled representatives from the federal agencies about weaknesses in the preliminary studies and the processes their agencies used to analyze the studies' conclusions and make decisions about how to proceed. The hearing followed a linear path, as witnesses built on testimony from the witnesses who preceded them, and concluded with an adversarial encounter with the agency officials. Waxman organized his witnesses into four groups, each offering a fundamentally different perspective on the issue and, like Scheuer, he concluded by calling to the table the group of witnesses he intended to interrogate most harshly: representatives of the aspirin industry.

The first group of witnesses that Waxman called represented the National Reye's Syndrome Foundation and consisted mostly of parents whose children had suffered from RS. Joel Taubin, a physician and vice president of the NRSF, and his wife briefly described how their eleven-year-old son suffered and died from Reye's syndrome. Taubin had heard about RS when he was a medical student, but "was told at that time by the department of pediatrics it is such a rare disease I will probably never see it." After their son died, the Taubins ardently sought answers to why and how he had contracted Reye's syndrome, asking "Was it something in our house, our environment?" Once the alleged link between aspirin and Reye's syndrome became known, Taubin threw his efforts into educating other parents about the potential threat. He concluded by thanking Waxman and the members of the subcommittee.

John and Terri Freudenberger, cofounders of the National Reye's Syndrome Foundation, followed the Taubins and told a similar story about the death of their daughter, Tiffini, in 1973 and their efforts to educate the public about the link between RS and aspirin. John Freudenberger, the president of the NRSF, described how, in the wake of Tiffini's death, they had built the foundation, which by 1985 had grown to 130 chapters in forty states. "We raise and provide money for two purposes: One, to save lives through increased awareness, and number two, to eliminate Reye's syndrome as a medical problem through research."

Freudenberger testified that authorities had moved too slowly and too cautiously to recognize and prevent Reye's syndrome, and over the previous decade they had made mistakes that slowed progress in identifying, treating, and eliminating the cause of RS. In 1974, the National Institutes of Health had mistakenly delayed recognition of Reye's syndrome and refused to allocate research funding to it. Reye's syndrome was not, as the surgeon general had recently claimed, a "rare" disease; rather, it struck "all too frequently and often fatally." The Ohio study that implicated aspirin in Reye's syndrome was, he said, a "mistake in planning" and had resulted only because the CDC had money left at the end of a year that it needed to spend quickly. The Food and Drug Administration made similar mistakes when it yielded to the aspirin manufacturers who quite effectively exploited errors in the original study to prevent labeling regulations. In the intervening years, the aspirin industry had "formed an organization that they called the Committee on the Care of Children, to give themselves an anonymous and more credible platform to oppose aspirin's implications in Reye's syndrome." He praised Waxman and the subcommittee for "trying to avoid yet another fatal mistake." The two couples that represented the National Reye's Syndrome Foundation submitted a stack of documents to the subcommittee that described their foundation's efforts as well as the status of Reye's syndrome in the United States. It included maps showing reported cases of RS, details of reported cases in Ohio from the previous year, several bulletins and advertisements warning about the link between aspirin and Reye's syndrome, and the foundation's most recent newsletter.

The last two statements from the first group of witnesses were offered by parents whose children had recently been stricken with Reye's syndrome. Gail Happle described the death of her six-year-old daughter. Her testimony was brutal and raw—scarcely a month had passed since the child's death. George Dumigan, whose daughter had just come out of a six-week coma, told a similarly terrible story. Both parents blamed aspirin, and both asserted that they would never again give it to a child.

In the question and answer period that followed the parents' testimonies, two surprising issues emerged. The first came in an exchange between Waxman and John Freudenberger, the president of the NRSF. Waxman, having already seen the materials submitted by the day's witnesses, reported that later in the day he expected that the representative from the Aspirin Foundation would testify that a "Reye's parents' group" opposed the enactment of a law that would require warning labels on aspirin bottles. Freudenberger, who ardently supported the passage of such a law, explained that there were three different organizations in the United States that represented parents of children with Reye's syndrome. His organization—the National Reye's Syndrome Foundation—was the largest, and it had recently agreed to merge with the second-largest organization, the Reye's Syndrome Foundation of Michigan. The third, and smallest Reye's syndrome organization was based in Denver, and Freudenberger referred to it as "a small group [that] has always yielded to the Aspirin Foundation" because "they need the money of the Aspirin Foundation."

The second surprise that emerged from the first group of witnesses came when Scheuer took the floor. He did not bother to question any of the witnesses. Instead, he offered them his sincere appreciation and told them "how deeply touched" he was by their testimony. Scheuer's attack on the Department of Health and Human Services for their efforts to educate parents about aspirin and Reye's syndrome had taken place only two and a half years earlier, but Scheuer seemed to have completely reversed his earlier position. He told the grief-stricken parents that he believed that the notice did not go far enough and that it would have to be augmented by an aggressive public education campaign. Without Jonah Shacknai whispering in his ear, Scheuer's beliefs about the possible role of aspirin in the onset of Reye's syndrome appear to have changed considerably. There is little beyond Shacknai's departure from government service that explains why Scheuer's views changed so dramatically between 1983 and 1985. No new studies on the relationship between aspirin and Reye's syndrome were produced between the two hearings, and no new substantial evidence had emerged linking aspirin use to Reye's syndrome.

The second group of witnesses—representatives from Public Citizen and the American Academy of Pediatrics—turned the subcommittee's attention away from the children who suffered from Reye's syndrome and toward the potential causes of RS. Sidney Wolfe, the director of Public Citizen's Health Research Group, described his organization's legal efforts to compel the HHS to require warning labels on aspirin. By 1985, Wolfe and Public Citizen had been involved in this issue for about three years, and he testified that he was "getting sick and tired of hearing from the aspirin industry and from the government that there are flaws in the studies." The flaws, he said, were minor, and any cases of Reye's syndrome that resulted from children ingesting aspirin were the result of "flaws in the morals and ethics of . . . anyone . . . who participated in any way to block something that could have saved the lives of many children and prevented a lot of brain damage."

Wolfe was followed by Albert Pruitt, the chairman of the department of pediatrics at the Medical College of Georgia and chairman of the Committee on Drugs of the American Academy of Pediatrics. He described the state of scientific knowledge about the relationship between aspirin and Reye's syndrome in much less certain terms than the congressmen had used. The AAP was involved in an ongoing review of the data and expected to be able to make firm recommendations soon. However, there was already sufficient evidence of a possible causal link between aspirin and Reye's syndrome to warrant strong admonitions against giving aspirin to children with the flu or chicken pox. Waxman was even more direct in the question and answer period that followed Pruitt's prepared statement. He bluntly asked, "If my kids get sick during this flu season, should I give them an aspirin?" Pruitt replied, "No, sir."

By the end of Wolfe's and Pruitt's testimonies, an underlying theme emerged. Taubin, the physician vice president of the NRSF who had lost a son to Reye's syndrome, had earlier stated his concern about the overuse of medications to treat illnesses that would probably resolve without treatment. "We don't have to treat every symptom," he asserted. Pruitt reiterated and expanded on Taubin's concerns. "There are many, many times with most infectious illnesses, that are nonbacterial, the child probably doesn't need any medication. We overtreat fever. We overtreat other symptoms. I think this also provides us an opportunity to evaluate whether or not a medication is actually needed." His remarks were very much reminiscent of the message that emerged at the end of one of the medical journal's letters to the editor of *Pediatrics* written by Karen Starko and George Ray. In using aspirin and other pain relievers and antipyretics to treat minor illnesses, we might in fact be engaging in "overzealous therapy" that "may be deleterious to the patient."

Both of the first two sets of witnesses were asked to comment on the efficacy of the federal agencies' efforts to prevent Reye's syndrome by warning parents about a possible link between aspirin and RS. None of the witnesses believed that the voluntary labeling agreement was working, and some—especially Sidney Wolfe—were highly critical of the agencies' willingness to please aspirin manufacturers. "In summary," Wolfe had concluded, "the voluntary program is a cruel disaster." Wolfe's pointed criticism appears to have been entirely in line with Waxman's opinion of the agencies' actions, so the stage was well set when Waxman called representatives from the FDA and HHS to the witness table.

Frank Young, the commissioner of the Food and Drug Administration, offered a fundamentally different view of the scientific certainty about the alleged causal relationship between aspirin and Reye's syndrome in his prepared statement to the subcommittee. In contrast to the solid certainty of a link expressed by most of the previous speakers, Young asserted that "definitive scientific data are still not available." What was available, he said, was "highly suggestive," but the small size of the pilot study "means that its findings should not be considered definitive." As a result, "the evidence to support the mandatory labels is not in our view available at this time." He also offered an entirely different view of the role of the aspirin industry than that offered by witnesses like Wolfe. "We feel," he said, "that we have under the leadership of Secretary Heckler forged a significant degree of public/private sector cooperation that addresses both the short-term and the long-term considerations." He was, nonetheless, happy to hear how the agencies might improve their public education efforts.

In the question-and-answer period that followed Young's prepared statement, Waxman and several other congressmen were blunt in their criticism of agency officials. Waxman told Young, "Well, you are being awfully nice to the aspirin industry if you are concerned about their making sure they can sell the aspirin during the flu season without disturbing their profit picture." Similarly, Representative Ron Wyden of Oregon told him, "Dr. Young, you don't look like a callous man to me. . . . But the effects of these actions in my view are very, very callous."

The Aspirin Industry Testifies

The last set of witnesses in Waxman's hearing consisted of representatives of aspirin manufacturers and retailers, who had developed a set of arguments that responded to the alleged causal relationship between aspirin and Reye's syndrome. It began with Joseph White, the president of the Aspirin Foundation of America, who seized on many of the arguments that had already been offered in support of requiring labeling of aspirin bottles to argue precisely the opposite. Whereas the congressmen and many of the witnesses had argued that the evidence of a causal link between aspirin and RS was "strong and consistent" and thus "Congress must act," White insisted that legislators "listen to the scientific data," which were incomplete and included clues to suggest that aspirin was actually not the culprit. For example, he claimed, children with juvenile rheumatoid arthritis took aspirin in high quantities for many years and "have no more Reye's syndrome than other children." Similarly, he agreed with the witnesses who talked about how terrible an ailment Reye's syndrome was, but he asserted that it had "occurred in many children who have never been given aspirin," so by assuming that it was caused by aspirin it was possible that "this terrible disease will go on, and we will have to start out all over again and reinstitute the search for what is the real cause."

Despite White's claims, researchers had in fact found evidence that children who regularly received aspirin to treat juvenile rheumatoid arthritis did have higher rates of RS than did children who did not regularly receive aspirin. In February 1984, a full year before Waxman's hearings on Reye's syndrome, researchers from Pennsylvania State University's Milton S. Hershey Medical Center published an account of two children with juvenile rheumatoid arthritis and a history of aspirin consumption who had developed Reye's syndrome. Admitting that much more research needed to be conducted and that aspirin was an effective therapy for juvenile rheumatoid arthritis, the researchers had nonetheless supported the AAP's recommendations to avoid aspirin use in children during outbreaks of chicken pox or influenza. In the fall of 1985, six months after the hearing, a group of researchers in Michigan also produced evidence that showed a heightened incidence of Reye's syndrome among children with juvenile rheumatoid arthritis. They concluded, "These findings support previous studies that showed that the use of aspirin during the antecedent illness may be a risk factor for the development of RS."

James Cope took an even more confrontational approach to the proposed labeling law than did White. Cope was president of the Proprietary Association, a century-old nonprofit organization that represented manufacturers and distributors of nonprescription, over-the-counter medicines. His prepared statement to the subcommittee offered four arguments against requiring a strict warning label on aspirin bottles. First, he asserted that there was "disagreement among scientists" about whether or not aspirin was causally involved in Reye's syndrome. Second, the proposed label would legally require that the warning about Reye's syndrome supersede all the existing warnings that are voluntarily placed on aspirin-containing products. Third, labeling and the associated product advertising that would be required by the proposed law simply could not accomplish all that the legislators hoped to accomplish with it. Advertising is "extremely limited as to how much information it can effectively carry," and as "the information load increases, consumers are inclined to tune out or to form wrong impressions." Fourth, the proposed law would levy stiff penalties on the "tens of thousands of retail establishments, bars, restaurants, service stations, motels, hotels, which . . . sell small cartons of aspirin-containing products."

The third and final representative of the aspirin industry to testify was Neil Chayet, a lawyer who represented the Committee for the Care of Children, the industry-backed organization that had been created in 1982. Chayet was even more aggressive than was Cope in arguing against the proposed law. Like Cope, he asserted that "science does not support the warning, period." He called the early studies "disastrous" and claimed that the agencies themselves had "thrown out" three of the four. Finally, he disputed the claim that industry pressure had led the HHS to reverse its plans to order the labeling of aspirin bottles three years earlier. "It was because the science was not there, and a mistake was made," he declared. "[T]hat was why the Academy of Pediatrics recommended no relabeling of aspirin at that time, because the science wasn't there." The historical record demonstrates that in fact the evidence was there, but the aspirin industry had used legal threats to bully the AAP into withdrawing their initial recommendation.

The subcommittee hearing concluded just three hours after it began with a short question and answer period with the three industry representatives. Waxman and Wyden pressed them for a formal statement of their opinion on the alleged link between aspirin and Reye's syndrome. Each responded that he was unconvinced of a causal relationship given the evidence at hand. Waxman eloquently summarized the situation: "It seems to me that [it] is quite an amazing position for the Food and Drug Administration and the Department [of Health and Human Services] to take to let somebody who doesn't believe in a position be the one to communicate that position."

The hearing ended with a nasty exchange between Waxman and Chayet, the lawyer who represented the Committee on the Care of Children. Chayet declared, "If we ever found out that there was a relationship between Reye's syndrome and aspirin, we would be the first to be before you to say so, sir." Waxman replied coldly, "That is what they say in law school." Chayet responded by saying that he resented the comment, and Waxman said simply, "You have to make the best case you can."

The record of the hearing concludes exactly as it began, with a story of a child who suffered and died from Reye's syndrome. Included at the end of the formal record of the hearing was a handwritten letter from Edwin D. Wigutoff of Seacliff, New York. Two years earlier, his thirteen-year-old daughter had developed the symptoms of Reye's syndrome and died. The pain and confusion of her death was still evident in the four-page letter. Wigutoff described how his wife had given their daughter aspirin to combat a low-grade fever, which was quickly followed by the familiar symptoms of RS: listlessness, confusion, and delirium. They rushed the child to the hospital, but her symptoms continued, and she died two days later. Wigutoff concluded, "The real tragedy here is that certain information was available but not distributed and our child might still be alive if we had known." Waxman's hearing took place more than four years after Karen Starko and her colleagues first found indications of a link between aspirin and Reye's syndrome. For the Wigutoffs and other parents who lost children in the intervening years, the delay in informing them of the possible relationship seemed inexcusable.

Mandatory Labels

By the fall of 1985, nine months after it was announced, the voluntary labeling program had been declared inadequate, and calls for a mandatory labeling program resumed. Waxman called the voluntary label "one of the stupidest warning I'd ever seen" because "it communicates nothing to anyone." The label merely said, "Do not use in persons under 16 years of age with flu or chicken pox unless directed by your doctor," and it avoided identifying Reye's syndrome by name. The voluntary label had allowed the HHS to avoid OMB oversight on the issue, but it said nothing about a possible link between Reye's syndrome and aspirin. It told parents only that they should not give aspirin to children or teenagers without first consulting a doctor. Waxman lamented, "No one whose child has a fever is going to call a doctor in the middle of the night after reading that label. A parent will want to do something to reduce the fever and give the aspirin anyway—maybe with fatal results."

The new label, with stronger language and a direct mention of Reye's syndrome, seemed to face little opposition in the fall of 1985. Senators Orrin Hatch and Howard Metzenbaum announced that a consensus on the policy change had been reached among agency officials, and the regulation would go into effect the following spring and expire two years later unless it was renewed. The new notice would read: "WARNING: Children and teenagers should not use this medicine for chicken pox or flu symptoms before a doctor is consulted about Reye Syndrome, a rare but serious illness." The following spring, Otis Bowen, the new secretary of Health and Human Services (and the third consecutive HHS secretary to deal with this issue) announced the agency's final decision on the issue. Before the start of the next RS season, warning labels directly mentioning Reye's syndrome would appear on all bottles of aspirin sold in the United States.

So the political dispute over whether to label aspirin bottles ended in 1986, more than half a decade after Karen Starko and her colleagues first identified a relationship between aspirin and Reye's syndrome. But the fight over aspirin and RS was far from over.

CHAPTER NINE

Triumph and Dissent

By the mid-1980s, the reported incidence of Reye's syndrome had begun to decline—and decline quickly. Researchers noticed the trend, and after various epidemiologic studies, they attributed the falling rate to declining aspirin use. By 1986, the year that the FDA began formally requiring the labeling of aspirin bottles to warn about a possible association with Reye's syndrome, only a few dozen children were given diagnoses of RS. While health officials and epidemiologists maintained a high level of vigilance and continued to warn parents to watch for the symptoms of Reye's syndrome, they simultaneously began developing what I call a triumphalist narrative about the emergence of the aspirin hypothesis and the subsequent near-elimination of Reye's syndrome.

The triumphalist narrative about Reye's syndrome begins with descriptions of how thousands of children suffered from a mysterious illness and many died, and others were left permanently damaged. After physicians had developed diagnostic criteria and treatments to improve the prognosis of children diagnosed with RS, public health officials applied their tools to identify the cause of Reye's syndrome. They quickly narrowed their search to a culprit that seems to have always been near the bottom of the list of suspects: aspirin. After 1980, the worst year on record for reported cases of Reye's syndrome, public health researchers offered carefully worded explanations of their findings that strongly suggested a correlation between aspirin and Reye's syndrome. With the help of federal officials and despite resistance from corporate interests, warnings about administering aspirin to children were heeded by physicians and parents, and Reye's syndrome quickly disappeared even before researchers were able to develop their evidence of a correlation between aspirin and RS into a demonstration of a causal relationship. This triumphalist narrative first appeared in the late 1980s, and it has become increasingly compact. Today it is a textbook case of how science and public health policy can turn tragedy into triumph.

This triumphalist account of the discovery of the relationship between aspirin and Reye's and the subsequent demise of Reye's syndrome was repeated outside the United States. For example, as early as 1986 the United Kingdom's Committee for the Safety of Medicines published an update on Reye's syndrome that quickly summarized the evidence in favor of a correlation between aspirin and RS, then explained how the decline in cases of Reye's syndrome combined with the shortcomings of existing studies led to a situation in which a causal relationship could not be established. Nonetheless, the report strongly intimated a causal relationship based on the concurrent public education campaign, the decline in aspirin use, and the steep drop in the annual number of reported causes. The educational campaign that the FDA began in 1985 warned parents against giving aspirin to children with influenza or chicken pox. "Subsequently," the U.K. report concluded, "fewer children in the U.S. have received aspirin for these conditions and the numbers of reports of Reye's syndrome have declined substantially." Without explicitly stating a causal relationship between aspirin and Reye's syndrome, it is not at all unreasonable for a reader to conclude that there probably was a causal link.

There is good evidence to show that in fact aspirin use did decline throughout the same time that the cases of Reye's syndrome rapidly disappeared, so that part of the story is empirically supportable. Evidence of the decline in aspirin use came in 1986, when several of the Michigan researchers published a paper in *Pediatrics* that explored the frequency of aspirin use in children over the previous five years. They surveyed nearly two hundred families with young children in Tecumseh, Michigan, a community of about ten thousand residents in the southeast corner of the state. The researchers found that aspirin use there had fallen from about 56 percent to 25 percent among families with young children over the first four years of the 1980s. In addition to finding a significant increase in the percentage of parents who chose not to give their ill children any painkillers or antipyretics, they found that the vast majority (90 percent) of the parents surveyed in 1983 knew that there was a possible association between aspirin and Reye's syndrome. Only 11 percent of the parents surveyed in 1983 reported that they had continued to give their children aspirin as frequently as they had five years before. The researchers believed that the decline in aspirin use among the families in Tecumseh could represent a nationwide decline in aspirin use in children, and they believed that the decline "most likely results from the widespread publicity about the association between aspirin and Reye syndrome." In the subsequent studies in Ohio and Michigan as well as the pilot study conducted by the U.S. Public Health Service, a small but statistically significant percentage of parents had stopped giving aspirin to their children.

The Michigan researchers found evidence that the aspirin hypothesis had caused a decrease in parents' use of aspirin, and they combined that conclusion with the documented decrease in the reported cases of Reye's syndrome to argue that their findings supported the validity of the aspirin hypothesis. Citing the *Morbidity and Mortality Report* in 1980 that first described the Arizona and Ohio studies and the first Michigan study, they asserted, "If it is assumed that using aspirin increases the likelihood for developing Reye syndrome then according to one estimate, 88% of cases of Reye syndrome may be attributable in part to salicylate use. Accordingly, a decrease in the frequency of aspirin use should produce an associated change in the incidence of Reye syndrome." Therefore, given the alleged association between aspirin and Reye's syndrome recorded in the late 1970s and early 1980s, followed by a substantial decrease in both the use of aspirin in children and the incidence of Reye's syndrome, the researchers were even more confident that there might be a causal relationship between aspirin and Reye's syndrome.

By the end of the century, however, the carefully worded claims of a correlation between aspirin and Reye's syndrome hardened into the claim that "the etiologic role of aspirin is now well known and Reye's syndrome had been virtually eliminated because parents stopped using aspirin to treat fever in their children." Therefore, all that was left to do was to continue to vigilantly discourage parents from ever giving their children aspirin.

Heroes and Villains

A critical part of the creation of a triumphalist narrative is the recognition of heroes to be celebrated and villains to be excoriated, or at least identified. Reye himself is a hero of sorts in many of the stories, and the attachment of his name to the disorder is a mark of respect. The few biographical details that are available about his life and work emerge from his obituaries, which always tend extol their subjects' better qualities and minimize or ignore their faults. The most detailed obituary of Reye described him as an "extremely thorough" researcher who "pioneered" some of the studies he pursued, and it explained he was "shy and retiring," and "extremely helpful in his advice but on a personal level a delightful friend with his own brand of whimsical humour." Even articles that focus on the ailment itself tend to lionize Reye as "meticulous" and reluctant about publishing his early findings, which reinforces the image of Reye as a careful researcher who was not interested in whatever fame might come from identifying a new ailment.

Likewise, the physicians—often identified by name—as well as the many unnamed nurses who cared for the children suffering from Reye's syndrome throughout the 1970s sometimes emerge as heroes in the fight against the mysterious ailment. Nowhere was this more clearly seen than in the 1976 WBBN news story about the efforts to treat children with Reye's syndrome at the Cincinnati Children's Hospital. It showed physicians and nurses thoughtfully and gently caring for children suffering from RS, and calm and authoritative statements from physicians were followed by heart-wrenching images of sick children. The doctors' pitch for increased funds for research on Reye's syndrome augmented descriptions from the narrator about how long and hard the doctors fought to save their patients' lives.

All of the officers of the Epidemic Intelligence Service and their other colleagues employed by the CDC and state departments of public health are acknowledged for their work in crafting methods for elucidating the association between aspirin and Reye's syndrome. Among the CDC's EIS officers, Lawrence Schonberger is frequently identified for his work guiding the various state studies and directing vital resources into them. Likewise, Karen Starko, the lead author on the Arizona study, has sometimes emerged as a hero for first identifying a possible relationship between aspirin and Reye's syndrome. The height of their recognition in the published literature came in 2010 with the publication of Mark Pendergrast's *Inside the Outbreaks: The Elite Medical Detectives of the Epidemic Intelligence Service*. Behind a comic book–style cover is a catalog of stories of the work of the EIS. "Because," Pendergrast explained, "public health efforts like those of the EIS are largely invisible—few people know they are being protected—they are both undervalued and underfunded, despite their efficiency."

Admiration for the public health researchers who studied Reye's syndrome is perhaps best seen in the occasional publications and the Web presence of the National Reye's Syndrome Foundation (NRSF), which still continues to function years after the annual number of reported cases has fallen to near zero. Take, for example, the publication produced for the NRSF's thirty-fifth anniversary and dedicated to "the many who served . . . The many who made a difference . . . The many who lost children and turned around and saved other children . . ." The coffee-table book begins with a timeline of the discovery of RS and the organization's evolution, and it ends with a long section of biographies of children who had contracted Reye's syndrome, many of whom had died. In between is a catalog of physicians and researchers who are recognized for their contributions to the study of the illness.

The identification of villains appears to be every bit as important to the triumphalist narrative of Reye's syndrome as has been the recognition of the story's heros. In the popular depictions of RS that began to appear in the early 1970s, the ailment itself is the enemy. Anthropomorphized as a mysterious killer, the nearly two-decades-long struggle to understand its cause and develop treatments for it reads like a murder mystery.

But in the earliest public depictions of Reye's syndrome we see that the ailment itself was not the only villain in the story. Just as Rachel Carson's *Silent Spring* established the script for discussions about health and the environment throughout the 1960s, early suspicions that Reye's syndrome was caused by spraying for spruce budworm instituted a narrative about greedy companies buying politicians' votes. The forestry companies and the political leaders from the Canadian provinces whose economies depended upon them were frequently identified as bad guys in the Reye's syndrome story. The Canadian politicians' unwillingness to accept Crocker's conclusions about the relationship between spraying and Reye's syndrome instigated criticisms from the public that politicians were willing to allow children to die in order to keep lumber mills stocked with wood.

The physicians who were involved in the research on Reye's syndrome and active in treating children afflicted with it also pointed fingers at politicians. As early as the mid-1970s, accounts of RS appeared that focused on inaction in Washington as contributing to the deaths of children from the mysterious illness. Again, nowhere was this clearer than the 1976 news story about the Cincinnati Children's Hospital. The announcer proclaimed, "Doctors here who work 16 to 20 hours a day trying to save children's lives complained that there is no willingness to devote more federal money for research into childhood diseases." The accusation that politicians and agency bureaucrats were slow to institute labeling fits nicely into the triumphalist narrative.

Once evidence emerged late in 1980 that there might be a relationship between aspirin and Reye's syndrome, federal agencies considered labeling aspirin bottles, and the narrative about Reye's syndrome slowly shifted to focus on the aspirin manufacturers' political efforts in the early 1980s. Lately, pharmaceutical companies more generally have received criticism for obstructing regulators' efforts, which aligns well with a growing public animosity toward the companies that had emerged in the 1990s. Of course, the problem with accusing pharmaceutical companies for slowing the labeling process is the fact that it really was only a small portion of the industry that was fighting to preserve aspirin's marketshare. The companies that manufactured acetaminophen and ibuprofen products kept quiet during these deliberations, as admonitions against using aspirin in children with viral illnesses would have only helped improve their products' share of the market.

The height of the triumphalist narrative about the disappearance of

Reye's syndrome came in 1999 with a paper in the *New England Journal of Medicine* that reviewed the decline of cases throughout the 1980s and 1990s and an accompanying editorial trumpeting the near demise of RS. Half a dozen researchers at the Centers for Disease Control authored the article, among them Lawrence Schonberger, who had led the CDC's surveillance of Reye's syndrome as well as the effort that eventually identified aspirin's association with the ailment. The "precise cause" of Reye's syndrome, they said, is unknown, but studies showed a "strong epidemiological association between ingestion of aspirin during the antecedent varicella or influenza-like illnesses and the subsequent development of Reye's syndrome." Salicylates were the only possible causal factor for RS that was suggested. By the late 1990s, when the paper was published, public health officials and epidemiologists were in a position to offer a retrospective analysis of the rise and fall of Reye's syndrome, chronicling both the nature of the illness and its victims. The researchers reported that between 1980 and 1997, the voluntary surveillance system had recorded 1,207 cases of Reye's syndrome in children under eighteen years of age. After 1994, there were no more than two cases of RS reported each year. Most of the 1,207 reported cases (92.6 percent) had occurred in white children, and slightly more than half of the cases were girls. The majority of the children (93.1 percent) had experienced some sort of prodromal illness of either a respiratory infection or chicken pox (there were about three cases of respiratory illness for every one case of chicken pox). Cases appeared in a particular season each year, from December through April, mirroring the influenza season. Before 1990, the incidence of Reye's syndrome was higher in the years that saw a higher number of cases of influenza B than in years during which influenza A was more common. This pattern, however, fell away after 1990, when the number of cases reported annually dropped to a mere handful.

The entire discussion section of the paper focused on the relationship between aspirin and Reye's syndrome, and there was a strong intimation that the decline of Reye's syndrome was causally related to the recognition of aspirin's relationship to the ailment. After peaking at 555 in 1980, the number of cases reported annually to the CDC had fallen quickly over the next several years. "The decline," the authors asserted, "followed reports of the association of Reye's syndrome with the use of aspirin during an antecedent varicella and influenza-like illness." This decline, they concluded, "demonstrates the importance of disseminating timely preventative messages to the public."

The retrospective study of Reye's syndrome was accompanied by a celebratory editorial by Arnold Monto, a professor of epidemiology at the University of Michigan. Titled "The Disappearance of Reye's Syndrome—A Public Health Triumph," Monto's editorial compared the fear parents had about Reye's syndrome in the 1970s and 1980s with the fear their own parents had of polio. Both, he said, generated headlines in local newspapers and both could produce death or permanent disability in the afflicted children. Reye's syndrome, however, was not so easily recognized clinically as was polio, nor was it easily associated with a particular viral cause. The comparison of RS and polio allowed Monto to leverage the widely acknowledged success of the polio campaigns to generate an appreciation for the public health success that he believed the defeat of Reye's syndrome likewise represented. The demise of Reye's syndrome, Monto concluded, "should be recognized as the success that it is. This success story was the result of collaboration between the biomedical groups that conducted the critical studies and a public committed to preventing a dangerous disease in children." Future successes could therefore be achieved only with proper funding and a similarly compliant public.

On the heels of the retrospective article and the accompanying editorial, the *New York Times* published an account of the history of Reye's syndrome. Titled "A Tale of Triumph on Every Aspirin Bottle," it is the ultimate expression of the victory of the aspirin hypothesis and the struggle to protect children from a deadly ailment. So, by the turn of the century—less than forty years after Reye's syndrome was first described as a new "clinicopathological entity"—a triumphalist narrative had been established of its study, treatment, and elimination. Over the next several years, parts of that story would become increasingly useful in the hands of authors who wanted to demonstrate how politics could slow or even halt this process. By chronicling the many children who were disabled or killed by Reye's syndrome while lobbyists lobbied and politicians politicked, advocates for science had a powerful story about the need to prevent science from being politicized.

I began writing this book with a great deal of suspicion of the triumphalist narrative about aspirin and Reye's syndrome. It seemed too simple an explanation, one that left far too many questions unanswered. Why, for example, did we not see cases of encephalopathy and fatty liver in the medical literature before 1950? Why did Reye's syndrome appear so suddenly in the second half of the twentieth century in so many different countries around the world? And, equally curious, why did RS disappear in the 1980s, even in countries where aspirin consumption was always quite low? Shortly after I began this project I discovered James Orlowski's work—which stands in such sharp contrast to the triumphalist narrative about aspirin and Reye's syndrome—and I thought that perhaps I had discovered an explanation for Reye's syndrome far better than the one advanced by advocates of the aspirin hypothesis. I also thought that Orlowski's hypothesis might explain my own experience with RS.

A Catch in the Reye

Throughout the rise of the aspirin hypothesis and the establishment of the triumphalist narrative, one person—James Orlowski—has consistently undermined both. Orlowski had testified in the 1982 congressional hearing that Jonah Shacknai had so carefully orchestrated, and his qualifications to speak on the subject were difficult to undermine. Orlowski had first appeared in the medical literature on Reye's syndrome in 1979 when he was a physician at the pediatric intensive care unit at the Rainbow Babies and Children's Hospital in Cleveland, Ohio. As one of the states that saw especially high numbers of cases of Reye's syndrome in the 1970s, Ohio had been home to a great deal of activity related to RS, including the National Reye's Syndrome Foundation, one of the earliest epidemiological studies on RS, and the medical team led by William Schubert at the University of Cincinnati College of Medicine that had done much to advance treatment of Reye's syndrome. Orlowski appears to have developed an interest in Reye's syndrome in the late 1970s, and he continued to publish papers on it throughout the next three decades.

Orlwoski's first publication on Reye's syndrome described three cases with symptoms that were indistinguishable from RS, "but associated with elevated cold-agglutinin titers and antiglobulin-I autoimmune hemolytic anemia." That is, the children appeared to have Reye's syndrome, but their blood work indicated that they suffered from an autoimmune disorder that caused high concentrations of antibodies that attacked their red blood cells and caused anemia, which was not typically seen in patients with Reye's syndrome. Orlowski and two colleagues from the Rainbow Babies and Children's Hospital described the three cases, all with different outcomes despite similar courses of treatment. They had treated an eleven-month-old boy with five exchange transfusions along with phenobarbital therapy and dexamethasone and mannitol. The boy was put on a respirator and a feeding tube was inserted to keep him alive. He fell into a coma and was eventually transferred to a chronic care facility in a vegetative state. The second case involved a sixteen-month-old girl, who was likewise treated with exchange transfusions, mannitol, and dexamethasone. She slowly recovered, was released from the hospital a month later, and returned to health with no apparent neurological or developmental abnormalities. The third case was a seven-year-old boy, who received exchange transfusions every eight hours for two days and died after two more days of mannitol therapy.

Both the symptoms and the laboratory findings for all three children were consistent with Reye's syndrome, which by the late 1970s had been clearly defined. All three patients had prodromal upper respiratory tract infections followed by an apparent recovery before the onset of vomiting and deranged mental states that indicated encephalopathy. The children had been delirious before becoming unresponsive and falling into comas, all of which followed the clinical path that Reye had described fifteen years earlier. Their laboratory results showed them progressing through the stages of Reye's syndrome that Lovejoy had established, but also showed that the children had a particular autoimmune disorder that led to anemia. The additional feature of their patients' illnesses led Orlowski and his colleagues to consider their condition "a unique encephalophatic condition" that had not been previously reported in any of the literature. The paper received no published reactions, and it appears to have been cited only once, which was in a comprehensive review of Reye's syndrome that was published in 1981 in the *Canadian Medical Association Journal.*

Orlowski continued treating about ten patients with Reye's syndrome a year into the early 1980s, and he published three more articles on RS throughout the first years of that decade. In 1980, he joined three other physicians from the hospital's pediatric and surgical intensive care unit to publish a piece that was provocatively titled "Reye Syndrome: A Predictably Curable Disease." Orlowski and his colleagues summarized the previous decade's publications on protocols for treating Reye's syndrome and emphasized that "the most important factor in the successful management of Reye syndrome is the early identification of its victims and the institution of aggressive therapy as early as possible" to prevent the children's symptoms from progressing to more serious stages. This would require "family practitioners and pediatricians to have a high index of suspicion and be willing to diagnose Reye syndrome provisionally on the basis of a history of recent viral infection and persistent vomiting, sleepiness, lethargy, or combativeness." Treatment, they asserted, should focus on two primary issues: supportive therapy such as mechanical respiration or sedation and management of the patients' growing intracranial pressure with hypothermia, hyperventilation, and drugs. Ultimately, the article represented an attempt to accept Reye's syndrome as inevitable given the current state of knowledge about its causes and to treat it as aggressively as possible to prevent children's symptoms from growing more severe. The next two pieces that Orlowski published in the early 1980s on Reye's syndrome both appeared in the *Cleveland Clinic Quarterly* and focused on tactics used to maintain acceptable intracranial pressures in patients with Reye's syndrome. Both described particular cases, the attempted therapies and the outcomes. These two articles demonstrated Orlowski's commitment both to treating patients afflicted with RS and in advancing the state of medical science. Given their publication in low-profile journals and their very low citation rate in subsequent papers on RS, they appeared to have had little impact on the discussion.

In 1984, Orlowski published his first article that openly questioned the alleged relationship between Reye's syndrome and aspirin, and he continued to publish criticisms of the aspirin hypothesis for nearly twenty years. While he never claimed that there was *no* relationship between RS and salicylates, he resisted what he believed was a hasty adoption of the aspirin hypothesis that had caused the public and professional conversation to depict aspirin as *the* cause of Reye's syndrome. He asserted that the correlation between aspirin and RS did not mean there was a causal relationship, and he feared that the medical community would lose a valuable tool in treating childhood illness if aspirin were wrongly implicated in causing Reye's syndrome.

The first published statement from Orlowski that reflected his concerns about the aspirin hypothesis came in his letter to the editor of the *Journal of the American Medical Association* in 1983 and focused on the quality of the data that had been used in the study by the Ohio Department of Health. He wrote to say that he was "somewhat confused" by the data presented in an article in the journal a few months earlier that had described its finding that ninety-four of the ninety-seven children with Reye's syndrome in the study had reportedly used aspirin, while only 110 of the 156 controls with RS had reported taking it. The authors of the paper had concluded, "This study shows that aspirin at normal doses is associated with RS."

Orlowski explained in his letter that his institution had participated in the Ohio study and that he had reported five cases of Reye's syndrome to the Ohio Department of Health and that only two of those patients had received aspirin. "I find it hard to believe," he wrote, "that two of the three patients with Reye's syndrome who had no history of aspirin ingestion were from a single institution, namely, the Cleveland Clinic." Moreover, it appears that another patient he had reported with Reye's syndrome that had not ingested aspirin was excluded. Orlowski concluded by asserting that the discrepancies between what he reported and the data used in the study "raises questions as to how cases were selected for inclusion in the study (that is, selection bias), assuming that there was no breakdown in the reporting mechanisms."

The authors of the Ohio study responded to Orlowski's concerns, saying that they had in fact received reports of only two cases of Reye's syndrome from the clinic at which Orlowski worked during the study period, and one of them could not be adequately verified, so it was excluded. A total of thirty-three hospitals had reported cases, and the authors stated that there was "no evidence of similar reporting problems at the other 32 hospitals." They admitted to an error, which had been reported in a previous issue of the journal that had caused them to overlook the one patient Orlowski reported with Reye's syndrome who had not taken aspirin. They responded to Orlowski's allegations of selection bias by saying it had "no foundation." The nurses who had coordinated the study, they stated, "were not only entirely unaware of the possible association between aspirin and Reye's syndrome, but had no information concerning medication use before the enrollment of cases and control in this study."

The following year, Orlowski used the same tactic—a letter to the editor expressing confusion with a published claim about the aspirin hypothesis—in response to a paper published in the summer of 1983 in the *New England Journal of Medicine*. The paper in question had been written by a team of physicians at Cincinnati Children's Hospital and had used data that had also been included in the Ohio study and published in the *Federal Register*. Orlowski had written to question the details of the thirty-one patients who had taken aspirin, asking which ones had developed the most severe symptoms. By his calculations, the children that had taken aspirin experienced far less serious symptoms (never progressing past Lovejoy's stage I). He concluded, "If this is true, then salicylates may protect patients with Reye's syndrome from progression of their disease to more severe states." The two lead authors of the paper—Phillip Lichtenstein and James E. Heubi—responded by stating that between 75 percent and 100 percent of the children with more severe symptoms in fact had taken aspirin. "With this information available," they concluded, "it is apparent that salicylates confer no protection against disease progression in patients with Grade I Reye's syndrome."

That same year—1984—Orlowski published a systematic review of the evidence supporting an association between aspirin and Reye's syndrome in the journal *Postgraduate Medicine*, whose audience was mostly primary care physicians. Orlowski reviewed the symptoms and provided a thorough description of the state of knowledge on RS before explaining the results of the Arizona, Michigan, and Ohio studies. The bulk of the article consisted of an identification of flaws in the studies and an argument against requiring warning labels on aspirin. The studies, he said, suffered from problems with parental recall because the parents "of Reye's syndrome patients were under a great deal of stress, which would understandably affect their recall." There was also a lack of confirmation of the medications that children actually received, which was important because the "tendency of parents to refer to acetaminophen as 'liquid aspirin' raises an obvious problem in this regard." In point of fact, in the second Michigan study the researchers had actually examined bottles of every medication given to children during their prodromal illness. Orlowski also asserted that because more than 80 percent of the patients in the studies did not have liver biopsies, there is significant uncertainty about whether or not all of them actually had Reye's syndrome. Finally, there was the problem of case-selection bias, which Orlowski had already made public. Orlowski worried that, while medical professionals were well versed in the differences between a reported *cause* and an *association*, "the public, as a rule, is not and therefore will assume that a reported association between salicylates and Reye's syndrome means that aspirin causes Reye's syndrome." He asserted that aspirin is "an unlikely cause" of RS because it had been used for many years before Reye's syndrome was identified. Moreover, he argued, Reye's syndrome is both geographically and racially concentrated, whereas aspirin use is not. Orlowski argued against labeling because it would discourage the use of a drug that had proven benefits in the treatment of fever, pain, and inflammation, and it would probably be replaced with acetaminophen, which was too easily overused and quite dangerous. Most significant, he concluded, "the proposed labeling would prevent conduction of a proper prospective study or a well-performed case-control study on the question of salicylates and Reye's syndrome."

Orlowski published his most widely read—and most widely criticized—article on Reye's syndrome in 1987, after he returned to Australia to work with two colleagues studying the relationship between

Reye's syndrome and aspirin. With the clever title "A Catch in the Reye," Orlowski and his coauthors searched the medical records of the Children's Hospital in Camperdown, Australia and located twenty of them between 1973 and 1982 that fit the CDC's criteria for Reye's syndrome. Of the twenty, eighteen of the affected children had either a liver biopsy or an autopsy confirming the diagnosis of RS, which was the gold standard for diagnosing of the disorder. In Australia, aspirin was typically not given to children; instead, acetaminophen was the drug of choice for relieving children's pains and reducing their fevers. So it was not surprising that "only one child had ingested aspirin or salicylate-containing products, and this child had been vomiting repeatedly and had a zero salicylate level on admission to the hospital." They concluded, "It is difficult to reconcile this lack of association between aspirin use and Reye syndrome in Australia with the strong and statistically significant associations reported by the United States and individual state public health services." His only explanation for the stark difference was a number of faults he found with the U.S. Public Health Service studies.

Several critical letters followed the publication of "A Catch in the Reye," which collectively demonstrated how seriously proponents of the aspirin hypothesis took Orlowski's criticisms even as they assertively rejected them. Orlowski responded to each and every one. Harry McGee (one of the authors of the second Michigan study) and Dean Sienko of the Michigan Department of Public Health wrote to point out the different methodologies employed in the various studies and to note the significant difference in the median age of patients. The average age of children in Orlowski's study was less than two years of age, while the average age in the Arizona study was 12.1, and in the second Michigan study it was 10.2. The significant age differences raised questions of differences in the presentation and outcome of Reye's in infants and toddlers as compared to older children. Orlowski argued the significance of the difference in ages and suggested that if anything it would "have the obvious effect of increasing the apparent association with salicylates, because liquid aspirin is not available and infants and young children would not be able to take aspirin." A much longer and more detailed response to Orlowski's "A Catch in the Reye" came from Susan Hall of the Communicable Disease

Surveillance Centre of Britain's Public Health Laboratory Service. Her American counterparts at the CDC in Atlanta also offered a similarly dismissive response to Orlowski's claim.

Orlowski's views on Reye's syndrome culminated with two publications around the turn of the century that attempted to shift the explanation for RS away from the aspirin hypothesis and onto another possible cause. The first—"Whatever Happened to Reye's Syndrome? Did It Ever Really Exist?"—argued that Reye's syndrome was actually caused by a number of different metabolic disorders that exhibited similar symptoms. He identified forty-nine patients who had been given a diagnosis of Reye's syndrome in the 1980s, twenty-six of whom had survived. The surviving patients were tested, and fifteen of them were found to have inborn errors of metabolism, such as medium-chain acyl-CoA dehydrogenase deficiency (MCADD) or a urea enzyme deficiency. After studying the medical records of the twenty-four patients who had died, Orlowski and his colleagues found that almost all of them—86 percent—had metabolic disorders of some sort. This meant that the symptoms the children exhibited had led incorrectly to diagnoses of Reye's syndrome; the children actually suffered from inborn metabolic errors, not RS. These disorders had been first discovered in the 1980s, and today infants are routinely tested for many of them. As a result, by the turn of the century—by which time diagnoses of Reye's syndrome had disappeared—the vast majority of cases of inborn metabolic errors were identified even before the children began exhibiting symptoms. Orlowski concluded, "The disappearance of RS worldwide is probably related more to the discovery of metabolic disorders that presented with the clinical and biochemical picture of RS than to warning labels and the reduced use of aspirin in children. Whether aspirin plays a role in the manifestations of these metabolic disorders is unknown, but aspirin is probably not a threat to the vast majority of the pediatric population that does not have an inborn error of metabolism."

Three years later, in 2002, with two of his colleagues from the University Community Hospital in Tampa, Florida Orlowski published his last major contribution to the study of Reye's syndrome. Most of the article consisted of a recapitulation of the discovery, clinical aspects, and epidemiological studies of RS, concluding with a roll call of the handful of studies that were not able to identify a relationship between aspirin and Reye's syndrome. The authors dismissed the claim that RS disappeared in concert with declining use of aspirin, arguing instead that "[A] careful examination of the incidence of Reye's syndrome over the 1970s and 1980s shows that Reye's syndrome was clearly disappearing before warning labels were instituted in 1986." They concluded, "The disappearance of Reye's syndrome was probably related to the discovery and ability to diagnose inborn errors of metabolism which mimicked Reye's syndrome clinically, biochemically, and pathologically." Unlike his earlier "A Catch in the Reye," Orlowski's later pieces attracted little attention and almost no criticism in the form of letters to the editor.

In many ways, Orlowski's work undermines the "us-versus-them" formulation of the relationship between the scientific community and aspirin manufacturers that is embedded in the triumphalist narrative. However, it can do so only if Orlowski himself was free of influence by the aspirin manufacturers. Others, like John Wilson and R. Don Brown of Louisiana State University's Medical Center in Shreveport, had been labeled "representatives of the aspirin industry" for publishing criticisms of the aspirin hypothesis after they had accepted money from an aspirin manufacturer. Their 1982 paper in *Pediatrics* had criticized the four state studies for "mismatching of the severity of prodromal (prehospitalization) illness" in comparing children with Reye's syndrome to the controls. In a footnote they had asserted, "If scientific data are to be used for decision making by the government–academic complex, then such data should be analyzed sufficiently to consider all reasonable interpretations." Therefore, it was their "duty as academic scientists to describe faults in the prevailing interpretation and to give a reasonable alternative interpretation." At the end of their paper was a short acknowledgement section that read simply, "This work was supported, in part, by Schering Plough Corp." Almost all other authors on the subject ignored their work, but it surely was part of the aspirin industry's arsenal in its lobbying efforts during those critical months in the fall of 1982.

For Orlowski to remain clear of allegations that he was in the pocket of the aspirin industry, he would need to be free from any support from them, and that generally appears to be the case. The only reference to outside funding that appears in his scientific articles was a statement that he had been the recipient of a World Health Organization Travel Fellowship. During the 1982 congressional hearing that lambasted the Department of Health and Human Services for its plan to mandate warning labels on aspirin bottles, allegations emerged that Orlowski had been in contact with representatives of the aspirin manufacturer Sterling Drug. In a signed letter to the subcommittee, Thomas Halpin, the chief of the Bureau of Preventative Medicine at the Ohio Department of Health and the lead author of the Ohio study, twice alleged that Orlowski had gone to Sterling Drug with evidence to support his allegations of selection bias in the Ohio study.

At the hearing, Orlowski testified that in fact he had not contacted the aspirin manufacturer with his concerns about selection bias in the Ohio study. Instead, he explained, "What happened was that, over the last eight to ten months, I have been quoted at least three times in the medical press as having stated that I felt that the data were at best tenuous and insufficient to make the degree of recommendations that were being made." At medical meetings, Orlowski said, he had stated that he did not believe "that the association was strong enough at this time to recommend that parents not give aspirin to children with flu-like symptoms or varicella." A representative of a pharmaceutical company approached him, he said, but he did not know which company. The representative asked Orlowski if he wanted help pursuing his claims of selection bias in the Ohio study, but Orlowski declined. After Halpin had ignored his concerns for some time, Orlowski submitted his letter to the editor of the *Journal of the American Medical Association*, and as a courtesy sent a copy to the drug company representative. I think it is safe to assume that Orlowski ended up in a hearing stacked with critics of the aspirin hypothesis after Shacknai had received his name from Sterling Drug because of this exchange. Unlike Wilson and Brown, Orlowski's critics cannot easily claim that he is profiting from his alliance with aspirin manufacturers. However, I am left wondering how Orlowski could have been in the dark about which company had employed the representative, given the fact that he was able to send the representative a copy of his letter.

In the end, Orlowski's criticisms of the aspirin hypothesis now seem to be largely ignored by authors who discuss the history of Reye's syndrome. Aside from the responses generated by his "A Catch in the Reye," most of his publications have seen relatively little citation and few responses. The aspirin hypothesis seems much more widely accepted than is Orlowski's claim that the children's symptoms resulted from inborn metabolic errors. For the more recent authors who critically discuss the politicization of science, Orlowski's explanation of Reye's syndrome would fundamentally undermine their assertions that the aspirin manufacturers inappropriately delayed the labeling of aspirin bottles to warn parents about a possible connection to Reye's syndrome.

CHAPTER TEN

The Politics of Public Health

I HAD ORIGINALLY FOUND Orlowski's arguments compelling and reasonable. This scientific rebel might have produced the answer to the mystery of Reye's syndrome and its rapid disappearance. He had laid out the aspirin hypothesis's shortcomings, aspirin's long history of safety, the surprisingly rapid decline of Reye's syndrome even before labels became mandatory, evidence from countries that did not use aspirin but that had similar experiences with the rise and fall of RS, and findings from his own research. He also presented an alternative explanation and supporting evidence that, at the very least, were plausible. Perhaps even more alluring to me was the way in which Orlowski came to look like an underdog in the dispute.

If Orlowski was right, his thesis would have practical consequences for those of us who had contracted and survived Reye's syndrome. Our illnesses might have been caused by undiagnosed inborn metabolic disorders, so even though we survived them, we would still have those disorders and presumably still suffer their consequences. The most common disorder that Orlowski found among survivors of Reye's syndrome was medium-chain acyl-coenzyme A dehydrogenase deficiency, commonly known as MCADD or MCAD deficiency. People with MCADD have a genetic disorder that prevents them from being able to break down medium-chain fatty acids into acetyl-CoA, which is a molecule the body uses in many of its biochemical reactions.

The effects of MCADD look a lot like Reye's syndrome. After a period of fasting—which would likely occur in the course of a viral illness—the body releases different types of fats to be metabolized and used as energy sources. People with MCADD are unable to metabolize some of the fats that are released, so unmetabolized medium-chain fats accumulate in their bloodstreams and they begin exhibiting symptoms of encephalitis, including confusion, lethargy, seizures, and coma. Death in these situations was common. MCADD disproportionately affects white children because it is most prevalent in people of northern European descent, like those who settled the Great Lakes area where Reye's syndrome was most frequently diagnosed throughout the 1970s. Treatment is relatively simple: avoid fasting and seek immediate medical attention when ill. Physicians began identifying individual children with MCADD using screening tests for newborns at about the same time that Reye's syndrome finally disappeared.

After reading Orlowski's arguments, I began to consider the possibility that the scar on my ankle was not the only vestige of childhood experience with Reye's syndrome. Perhaps the very cause of my brush with RS was still within me. Aside from the reported commonality of MCADD among survivors of Reye's syndrome, I had some evidence to suggest that I might have MCADD. Since the late 1990s, I had suffered from occasional migraines. One or two times a year I would be hit with a brutal headache, intense irritability, and lethargy. The episodes would last a day or two at the most and subsided after I ate and slept. The migraine drugs prescribed by my family doctor did nothing to prevent or treat them. Not only would MCADD explain the illness that had hospitalized me in the early 1970s, but it might also explain the intense headaches I occasionally experienced.

Medium-chain fats, the kind of fats that people with MCADD cannot break down, are largely absent from the human diet. The only foods that are rich in them are horse milk, coconut oil, and palm kernel oil. Before the 1990s, very few northern Europeans consumed any of these products, so the genetic error that arose (probably in northern Germany, where the incidence of MCADD is highest) was of little consequence. However, since the late 1990s, palm kernel and coconut oils have been increasingly used in a variety of processed foods. For someone who harbored undiagnosed MCADD, these newly introduced oils created a new source for the problematic medium-chain fats. As part of the effort to identify the cause of my migraines, I had recorded the foods I had eaten in the hours and days before onset of the headaches. Processed foods—like the kinds that included palm kernel and coconut oils—frequently appeared in my diet just before the migraines did. Perhaps Orlowski was right; maybe the illness that Dr. Musselman had diagnosed as Reye-Johnson syndrome was actually a metabolic crisis brought on by an undiagnosed inborn metabolic error.

The next step in testing Orlowski's argument (at least as far as my case was concerned) was to get myself tested to determine if I had MCADD. A child of the seventies, I had missed the routine screening of newborns that began in the 1990s, so I needed my family physician to order the test for me. After explaining the situation and seeing my decade-long history of occasional migraines, he ordered the test.

It took two weeks for the results to come back from the lab, and during the wait the conclusion for this book nearly wrote itself as I imagined how neatly the story would end if my test results were positive. So I felt somewhat disappointed when I learned that I did not have the inborn metabolic error. In addition to explaining the cause of my migraines and my experience with Reye's syndrome, a diagnosis of MCADD would have added a tiny bit of support for Orlowski's arguments about the true cause of the rise and fall of Reye's syndrome.

But, even if I—or anyone else who had been given a diagnosis of Reye's syndrome—later tested positive for an inborn metabolic disorder, Orlowski's claims would still be disputed. Proponents of the aspirin hypothesis had already laid the foundation for a strong argument against the claim that the symptoms associated with Reye's syndrome were caused by illnesses like MCADD. Nowhere was this as clear as it was in the retrospective analysis of RS that appeared in 1999 in the *New England Journal of Medicine*, which was written by some of the foremost authorities on Reye's syndrome. In the second paragraph of the article the authors admitted that "various inborn metabolic disorders . . . can present with manifestations that mimic those of Reye's syndrome, and clinical differentiation is often difficult." The paper's penultimate paragraph returned to the issue, asserting that inborn metabolic disorders "mimic" RS. This presentation of Orlowski's thesis—without ever mentioning him by name or citing him—made the triumph achieved by the advocates of the aspirin hypothesis effectively invulnerable to Orlowski's claims.

Undoubtedly, James Orlowski was right about at least some of the identified cases of Reye's syndrome; they were actually misdiagnosed cases of inborn metabolic disorders. But in the end I do not think it matters. Given both the ability of clinicians to distinguish children with disorders like MCADD from those who do not have any identifiable inborn errors of metabolism and the existence of RS among apparently otherwise healthy children, Orlowski's hypothesis is simply not accepted by the vast majority of authorities on this subject. Because Reye's syndrome has all but disappeared in the United States, the point is moot. At least it is moot to the physicians and nurses who treated the sick children, the epidemiologists who studied the disorder, and the public health officials who had to devise ways to respond to a scary and mysterious childhood illness. The disappearance of Reye's syndrome was a glowing silver lining nonetheless surrounded by a gray cloud; without any cases to investigate, physicians and epidemiologists could not determine with any certainly the cause or causes of the thousands of cases of RS that had appeared throughout the latter half of the twentieth century. And so our cravings for certainty are tempered by our appreciation for the disappearance of a terrible illness. But the evidence suggesting that there was a relationship between aspirin and Reye's syndrome is tremendously strong, and we can be thankful that the disorder no longer appears every winter.

Primacy and Politics

After all my research, I still cannot say with any certainty why Johnson's role in the identification of the syndrome faded from memory or why the disorder came to be known simply as "Reye's syndrome." But the question raises a number of issues about how we decide to recount the history of Reye's syndrome and how the debate over the possible relationship between aspirin and Reye's syndrome influences our memory of the two men's work. Reye's and Johnson's articles had been published within days of one another, each with equally informative data about the symptoms suffered by their patients and with similar evaluations of previous cases presented in their respective areas. Despite any arguments that might suggest that both men should share credit for first recognizing the ailment, the term "Reye's syndrome" first appeared in print in 1965. It was not until the mid-1970s that any author referred in print to the ailment as Reye-Johnson syndrome. However, my Mayo-trained doctor had said "Johnson-Reye syndrome" when he described the condition to my mother in 1972, and some of the publications that emerged from physicians and researchers at the Mayo Clinic suggest that the term had been in common use there in the late 1960s. Nonetheless, the official warnings that appeared in the mid-1980s against giving aspirin to children always called the disorder Reye's syndrome, and by the mid-1990s it was rare to see or hear it called anything else. So, Johnson's role in identifying the syndrome has been generally ignored.

Certainly Johnson's inability to publish his article in the *American Journal of Diseases of Children* might have had something to do with his relative obscurity. That journal's rejection of the paper and its subsequent publication in the *North Carolina Medical Journal* meant that it was read by relatively few people. The circulation of the *North Carolina Medical Journal* was far smaller than was that of the *Lancet*, where Reye and his colleagues published their work. But I cannot help also thinking that Johnson's later statements undermining the aspirin hypothesis had at least something to do with the fact that he has been largely ignored.

Harry McGee, one of the coauthors of the second Michigan study, suggested another possible explanation. There has long been some degree of tension between medically trained physicians and scientifically trained epidemiologists, and the twenty-year-long search for the cause or causes of Reye's syndrome exposes some of the friction that exists between them. Johnson himself was a physician, but by becoming a CDC Epidemic Intelligence Service officer, he effectively took up the tools and perspective of an epidemiologist in the 1960s. Compared to Reye, whose research on the ailment never took him outside of the hospital, Johnson's "shoe-leather epidemiology" had him chasing leads across North Carolina. However, by the time that the political deliberations over labeling were raging in the early 1980s, Johnson had long since left public health work to practice as a pediatrician in Fargo,

North Dakota (coincidentally, my hometown). When he testified at the 1982 congressional hearing, he did so very much as a pediatrician and in opposition to the claims about an alleged relationship between aspirin and Reye's syndrome.

The tension between physicians and epidemiologists that is in evidence in the history of Reye's syndrome was first visible to me in the research conducted by John Crocker, the Canadian physician and researcher who had developed evidence suggesting that spruce budworm spraying might be a cause of Reye's syndrome. The cases that appeared in the sprayed areas and his extensive laboratory research led him and his colleagues to claim that exposure to emulsifiers in the pesticides made typically nonlethal viruses very dangerous to some children. When they pressed public health officials and elected political leaders to curtail the spraying, epidemiologists were engaged to determine if there was any evidence to support the theoretical potential of the sprays to cause Reye's syndrome. Walter Spitzer, chair of the department of epidemiology and health at McGill University, headed the investigation that eventually examined over three thousand charts and found "no geographic or temporal association were evident between exposure to the spray used for controlling spruce budworm in New Brunswick and the occurrence of Reye's syndrome." Moreover, they could find no difference in the frequency of cases of Reye's syndrome during years of heavy spraying as compared to years in which there was less spraying.

In Canada, the epidemiologists' conclusions effectively undermined Crocker's findings and his efforts to curtail the spraying programs, demonstrating the power of epidemiologists to declare authoritatively that a lack of correlation meant that there could be no causative relationship between a suspected factor and the onset of Reye's syndrome. In a similar fashion, the SEATO researchers' work in Thailand in the early 1970s was summarily dismissed when, years later, epidemiologists could find no evidence of a correlation between high levels of aflatoxins in food and increased incidences of Reye's syndrome. A lack of correlation meant that the epidemiologists could simply state that there was no basis for claiming a possible causative relationship. As the aspirin hypothesis rose to prominence in the early 1980s, the tables turned and physicians increasingly argued that while the Epidemic Intelligence Service officers had found evidence of a correlation between aspirin and Reye's syndrome, they had not established a causative relationship.

Perhaps nowhere in the history of Reye's syndrome was the tension between physicians and epidemiologists more evident than in some of the presentations made at the 2009 meeting of the National Reye's Syndrome Foundation. Lawrence Schonberger of the CDC, who had been an EIS officer in the early 1970s and had helped guide the work done by EIS officers to identify possible factors in the emergence of symptoms associated with Reye's syndrome, summarized the CDC's surveillance of RS and the collaborative work done to identify the "probable etiological role of aspirin for this terrible illness." In the middle of his nearly twenty-minute presentation, Schoenberger seemed to depart from his telling of the story of Reye's syndrome to describe the nature of the "art of epidemiology." He said, "My own experience with Reye's syndrome brought forth the tensions that exist between the central purpose of epidemiology and the translation challenge of having epidemiological results change public policy to improve health." I later came to understand that what had first appeared to be a tangent in his talk was in fact the very heart of his presentation, and it nicely demonstrated the difference in approach of epidemiologists as compared to physicians.

Although of significant importance to each other, epidemiology is an approach to improving the public health that is fundamentally different from a physician's efforts to improve an individual's health. Epidemiologists design studies that, from the start, are intended to inform policy decisions and to aid in the prevention of disease and harm or to identify the proximate and ultimate sources of illness or injury. As such, the framing of their research questions are shaped to no small degree by an understanding and appreciation of the governing bodies they seek to inform and influence. This approach contrasts with mainstream medicine, which primarily focuses on the art and science of healing of individuals and typically only secondarily on prevention. The differences between the two are what made the competing testimonies offered by physicians and epidemiologists at the 1980s congressional hearings so easy to place in opposition to one another. They also help us uncover and understand some of the complexity that exists in the politics of public health.

In 1983, after the first congressional hearing, and while advocates of the aspirin hypothesis were trying to develop a coordinated response to the aspirin industry's efforts to avoid labeling, a new claim emerged that undermined both Reye's and Johnson's primacy. Thomas Weller, a physician at the Harvard School of Public Health, published a two-part article summarizing the state of knowledge on chicken pox and shingles that included a short section exploring the relationship of these disorders to Reye's syndrome. Reye, he believed, should not be credited with discovering the syndrome that eventually bore his name. Instead, he asserted, "The 'Mortimer-Lepow syndrome' would be an appropriate eponym." In April 1962—a year and a half before Reye's or Johnson's paper appeared—Mortimer and Lepow had published an article in the *American Journal of Diseases of Children* describing four cases of children with dangerously low blood-sugar levels and presenting evidence that their conditions might have been related to their ingestion of aspirin. The symptoms exhibited by the four children that Mortimer and Lepow described looked a great deal like the symptoms that were commonly associated with Reye's syndrome. Weller's suggestion received a sharp reply from Reye's coauthor, James Baral. In a letter to the editor of the *New England Journal of Medicine*, Baral explained that at least eleven of the twenty-one children Reye treated had taken aspirin before the onset of their more serious symptoms, and their paper had reported that fact. Moreover, Baral said, Reye had treated his first child with the syndrome in 1951, which was a full decade before Mortimer and Lepow had seen their first case.

The suggestion that Mortimer and Lepow deserve credit for identifying the disorder that came to be called Reye's syndrome engages some of the same issues that undermine Johnson's case for it—but from the opposite direction. Whereas Johnson argued against the aspirin hypothesis, Mortimer had always been a proponent of it. In 1982, he was a member of the American Academy of Pediatrics Committee on Infectious Diseases, which concluded that "there is high probability that the administration of aspirin contributes to the causation of Reye syndrome." He had very publicly resigned when the AAP had momentarily capitulated to the aspirin industry's demands for more research before parents were advised not to administer aspirin to children. That same year he published an opinion piece in the *International Journal of Epidemiology* arguing that the warning against administering aspirin to children with viral illnesses was "the only prudent course of action." In 1987, he published another editorial, this time in the *Journal of the American Medical Association*, which reiterated justifications for the warning and attacked the aspirin manufacturers for taking an "adversarial position" on the issue. Finally, in 1990, he published a critical response to Orlowski's "A Catch in the Reye" with the similarly clever title "A Catch in the Reye Is Awry." For advocates of the aspirin hypothesis, Mortimer is a more attractive candidate than Johnson or even Reye to support as the true discoverer of Reye's syndrome because of his efforts in the 1980s against the aspirin industry's stalling tactics.

Using the History of Aspirin and Reye's Syndrome

Since the turn of the century, the history of Reye's syndrome has attracted the attention of more than just clinicians, epidemiologists, and public health officials. In the wake of the 2000 presidential election, the history of Reye's syndrome was raised in allegations that scientific research was being inappropriately politicized. In the midst of a series of disputes during George W. Bush's presidency, Bush's political opponents charged that the administration had systematically ignored the American scientific community's advice on issues concerning health and the environment. The issues were politically polarized, as Democrats accused Republicans of turning their backs on science and being inappropriately influenced by both religion and industry. Books—some relatively objective, others highly partisan—appeared that explored the role of science in American politics. For many of their authors, Reye's syndrome was a perfect example of how politicians ignored science and put economic interests before the health and safety of American children.

Casting the history of Reye's syndrome as simply a contest between science and big pharma is made difficult by the fact that in the 1980s the aspirin hypothesis was used in a series of battles between competing pharmaceutical companies. The 1970s and 1980s had witnessed what has been termed "the aspirin wars," as manufacturers of over-the-counter products that contained aspirin, ibuprofen, and acetaminophen fought one another for market share. Even though the three drugs are chemically distinct from one another, they all relieve fever and pain equally effectively. Acetaminophen does not appear to reduce inflammation as well as aspirin and ibuprofen do in large doses, but it also does not appear to encourage stomach problems the way that aspirin and ibuprofen can. Their similarities and the tremendous size of the consumer market led to an aggressive advertising competition among a handful of pharmaceutical companies that eventually led to a series of accusations of false advertising, unfair business practices, and eventually court cases.

In the late 1970s, Tylenol was on its way to becoming the over-the-counter drug of choice for pain relief and fever reduction, and it had increasingly displaced aspirin as parents' choice for mildly ill children. In 1979, children's Tylenol alone had seized more than 40 percent of the market share, while Bayer aspirin and St. Joseph aspirin each had less than half of that. By the mid 1980s, Tylenol had almost two-thirds of the market while Bayer, and St. Joseph together had less than 15 percent. In the spring of 1985, American Home Products, which marketed several products that contained aspirin or ibuprofen, filed a lawsuit against Johnson & Johnson, which marketed Tylenol, alleging more than a hundred counts of false advertising. American Home Products was particularly irritated about a series of advertisements in medical journals and direct mailings to physicians that alleged that "up to ⅓ of newly diagnosed gastric ulcers may be related to aspirin therapy," so the company sued to force Johnson & Johnson to end the advertising campaign and pay $167 million in damages. Johnson & Johnson responded with a long list of counterclaims that included unfair competitive practices, poaching of key employees, theft of trade secrets, and false advertising.

As part of Johnson & Johnson's counterclaim, its lawyers contended that American Home Products acted too slowly in warning parents about aspirin's possible link to Reye's syndrome. By the mid-1980s, aspirin had lost a significant portion of its share of the analgesic market to Tylenol, but Johnson & Johnson asserted that Tylenol's sales would have increased even faster had American Home Products and other companies that sold aspirin added warning labels to their products sooner. Johnson & Johnson claimed $1.1 billion in lost sales from the delay in labeling aspirin. The complexity of the case and the tremendous sums of money associated with damages led Judge William C. Conner to split the trial into three parts, one to settle allegations of false advertising, one to examine the merit of the alleged association of aspirin and Reye's syndrome as well as the economic impact of delaying the adoption of warning labels on aspirin, and one to determine appropriate damage claims.

In the first of three decisions, Judge Conner concluded that both companies had published ads that contained false or misleading claims. Judge Conner, who was well known for using vivid language in his opinions, wrote, "Small nations have fought for their survival with less resources and resourcefulness than these antagonists have brought with their epic struggle for commercial primacy in the O.T.C. analgesic field." In the intensity of their fight, both American Home Products and Johnson & Johnson had made unqualified claims that could not withstand scrutiny. American Home Products had made misleading comparisons between ibuprofen and acetaminophen as well as false claims about Anacin-3. Johnson & Johnson misled customers with the claim, "You can't buy a more potent pain reliever without a prescription." Judge Conner determined that ibuprofen was sometimes "substantially more effective" than Extra Strength Tylenol. The judge also found that the ads Johnson & Johnson had placed in physicians' journals were misleading.

The second trial that resulted from allegations of misconduct hurled back and forth between American Home Products and Johnson & Johnson centered on the claim that American Home Products had inappropriately profited from the delay in the labeling of bottles of aspirin to warn parents against giving the product to children. The case would have been a good opportunity for a reasoned, systematic review of the evidence that aspirin actually caused or triggered the symptoms associated with Reye's syndrome, but it never came to trial. Judge Conner dismissed the suit in the fall of 1987 in part because Johnson & Johnson was a member of the Proprietary Association, the over-the-counter-drug manufacturer's trade group that had aggressively campaigned against warning labels on aspirin. The results of the first two trials led Judge Conner to throw out the damage claims leveled by both companies, but the legal bickering continued for years after the decision.

At the same time that aspirin was increasingly blamed for causing Reye's syndrome, its principal competitor in the market—Tylenol—was facing its own problems. In the fall of 1982, seven people in the Chicago area died after ingesting Tylenol capsules that contained fatal amounts of potassium cyanide. Within a month, there was a copycat crime in California: a nonfatal dose of strychnine appeared in tampered Tylenol capsules. This was followed by more than 270 different incidents of product tampering. Johnson & Johnson quickly pulled Tylenol capsules off the shelves, which represented a significant financial blow to the company because capsules accounted for about 40 percent of the brand's sales. Johnson & Johnson had invested tremendous amounts of money in advertising to establish Tylenol as a popular brand, and collectively Tylenol products accounted for 15 percent of Johnson & Johnson's profits. The original case remains unsolved, but it led to significant changes in safety standards for packaging in the food and drug industries with the introduction of tamperproof seals and indicators that showed if a package had been opened. Combined, the alleged links between aspirin and Reye's syndrome on the one hand and the threat of cyanide- or strychnine-laced Tylenol capsules on the other left parents increasingly wary about the methods available to them to treat common childhood illnesses.

By the 1990s, Tylenol had bested aspirin in the market, but its victory may well have come with other unforeseen consequences for children's health. In 1998, on the eve of the declaration that the defeat of Reye's syndrome was a public health triumph, a group of researchers led by Arthur Varner at the University of Wisconsin School of Medicine suggested that the increasing use of acetaminophen might have fueled a dramatic spike in asthma among children. Beginning in the 1980s, as parents abandoned aspirin in favor of acetaminophen, the rate at which asthma was diagnosed among children rose dramatically from 3.6 percent in 1980 to 5.8 percent in 2003 and had leveled off in the 1990s when acetaminophen use peaked. Over the next decade, nearly two dozen different studies supported their hypothesis.

In the fall of 2011, John T. McBride of the Department of Pediatrics in Northeast Ohio Medical University wrote in *Pediatrics*, "In my opinion, the balance between the likely risks and benefits of acetaminophen has shifted for children with a history or family history of asthma. . . . [W]e need further studies . . . not to prove that acetaminophen is dangerous but, rather to prove that it is safe." That same year, an editorial in the journal *Clinical & Experimental Allergy* bluntly asked, "Have the efforts to prevent aspirin-related Reye's syndrome fuelled an increase in asthma?" Their answer, apparently, was "maybe." They concluded by agreeing with many of the authors who had explored the subject, saying "[A] drug that is so commonly used from childhood throughout adulthood, including in pregnancy, and that has been associated in multiple studies with a common childhood disease causing a high social and financial burden, demands more definitive studies." Describing the shortcomings of previous studies of the possible link between acetaminophen and asthma, their analyses sounded a lot like the lamentations about the shortcomings of the four state studies on the possible relationship between aspirin and Reye's syndrome.

In the end, a careful study of the history of Reye's syndrome, aspirin, and the politics of public health makes evident our collective desire for certainty and our intense frustration with ambiguity, especially when it comes to our children's health. It demonstrates that calls for additional information do not inevitably produce the information that will generate certainty around issues as complex and as politically charged as Reye's syndrome. Therefore, increasing the number of voices or the number of methodological approaches to studying a problem does not necessarily induce certainty. The people who want to avoid the emergence of consensus call for additional research, the obvious solution to a scientific problem. So, ironically, the apparent advocates of research are actually trying to avoid the emergence of certainty and the enactment of scientifically informed policy. Obviously, as we saw with the two congressional hearings, open deliberation does not inevitably produce any clear level of certainty. None of the obvious solutions are sufficient to produce the level of certainty we crave.

It seems that our desire for certainty is best served by a concerted effort to produce and organize relevant new information and to construct a narrative that gives decision makers and leaders a mandate to enact policy. The aspirin industry's efforts in the early 1980s—led by people like Jim Tozzi and Joseph White—presented evidence and produced a narrative that could inspire a certain level of confidence that aspirin was safe. Their goal was obviously to stall government action in the face of emerging evidence that aspirin might be involved in the onset of Reye's syndrome. Competing evidence would not be enough to overcome their narrative. Instead, advocates of the aspirin hypothesis needed to craft an agenda for both additional research and for political advocacy that would effectively counter the aspirin industry's claims. They did not finally overcome the opposing narrative until Reye's syndrome itself had all but disappeared, leaving us with lingering uncertainty but no real need for additional new policies.

In the end, parents have to negotiate these uncertain waters. In the middle of the night, as their children's fevers spike and they reach into the medicine cabinet for relief, Washington politics, researchers' findings, and lobbyists' machinations are far away. All that is certain is that parents hope to do their best to protect and comfort their children, and all that scientists, physicians, and politicians can do is try to produce research, advice, and policies that give parents the best chance of preserving their children's health.

Acknowledgments

Even though there is often only one name on the cover, books are almost always the product of collaboration among many people, and this one is no exception. My colleagues at James Madison College and Lyman Briggs College at Michigan State University helped me think through many of the issues involved in this project. Sherman Garnett, my dean in James Madison College, pushed me to reach beyond the relatively narrow confines of academia with this book, and I owe him special thanks for giving me the freedom to speak to a broader audience. I must also thank fellow historian Mark McLaughlin for supplying me with some research material I could not have obtained without his help. Georgina Montgomery and Susan Stein-Roggenbuck deserve special recognition for their comments on the manuscript at various times throughout the writing process. Similarly, my colleagues Tobin Craig, John Jackson, Andrea Amalfitano, Libby Bogdon-Lovis, and Christian Young were valuable resources as I wrote this book, and I thank them all.

One the great pleasures in writing a history of a recent topic has been the opportunity to actually speak with some of my historical subjects. This project has given me the chance to talk with a number of people who played key roles in the history of Reye's syndrome, and their contributions helped me better understand this complex story. In this regard, I owe thanks to Karen Starko and Michael Thaler, who offered their expert advice. Likewise, Cathy Zraik of the National Reye's Syndrome Foundation was a valuable resource for me throughout the project. I am especially thankful to Harry McGee for lending his time, advice, and tremendous memory to me as I worked on this book. Harry met with me several times, read the entire first draft, and made pointed comments that helped me organize my thoughts and sharpen the details of this story.

Teachers often learn a great deal from their students, and that has certainly been the case with my collaboration with Nathan Praschan. We worked together—in class and out—for much of the time that Nathan was an undergraduate at Michigan State University. He helped me gather the materials at the start of this project and, as it matured, he helped me identify and explore many of the key issues involved in the history of Reye's syndrome. Much of what is written here was originally conceived in conversations with Nathan and is supported by material he helped me find.

In the midst of researching this project, I accepted a one-year fellowship with the American Association for the Advancement of Science to work at the National Science Foundation. My time in Washington gave me firsthand experience in the politics of American science and medicine that helped shape much of the latter half of this book. I owe special thanks to Julia Lane and Rebecca Rosen for teaching me so much about how Washington works and about the place of science and medicine in American politics (and, conversely, the place of politics in American science and medicine).

While I was living and working in Washington, I met Jonathan Moreno, a fine historian, philosopher, and bioethicist, who was generous with his time and advised me to consider publishing this book with a trade press rather than a traditional academic press. He also introduced me to his editor, Erika Goldman at Bellevue Literary Press. Erika is the type of editor I had always hoped to find: she helped me develop the narrative arc of my book and pointed me toward ways to tell this story. The style, structure, and contents of this book are powerfully influenced by her contributions to it. I would also like to thank the press's staff, who have been so helpful throughout the process of writing and publishing this book, and especially Nancy Brooks, who copyedited the manuscript and greatly improved it in the process.

My wife, Brie Largent, has been a constant, loyal, and patient supporter of my work. Her willingness and ability to put our family before all else is inspiring, and I could not enjoy the successes I have experienced in my personal and my professional life without her. Together with our children, Annabelle and Elsa, she is a constant reminder of the most important things in my life.

Finally, the story I tell about my personal experience with Reye's syndrome hints at only a small part of the tremendous gratitude I feel toward my mom, Elizabeth Largent. She has always been there for me, and I hope that by dedicating this book to her I can show some of my appreciation for all that she has done and continues to do for me.

Notes

Prologue

page

11 "Dr. Bernard Musselman and . . ." "'Doctors for Ogdensburg' Discuss M.D. Shortage," *The Post-Standard* (Syracuse, N.Y.) November 19, 1966: p. 27. "Bernard C. Musselman, M.D.; Revocation of Registration," *Federal Register* 64 (1999): p. 55965. "Anne McDonald Becomes Bride of Bernard Musselman," *Ogdensburg Advance-News* (Ogdensburg, NY) September 15, 1958.

12 "It is not surprising . . ." For evidence that physicians and researchers at the Mayo Clinic were attentive to Reye's syndrome (which they referred to as Reye-Johnson syndrome), see Alfredo Nicolosi, W. Allen Hauser, Leonard T. Kurland, and Ettore Beghi, "Reye's Syndrome: Incidence and Time Trends in Olmsted County, MN, 1950–1981," *Neurology* 35 (1985): 1338–1340.

13 "Today, all that remains . . ." Ermias Belay, Joseph Bresee, Robert C. Holman, Ali S. Khan, Abtin Shahriari, and Lawrence Schonberger, "Reye's Syndrome in the United States from 1981 Through 1997," *New England Journal of Medicine* 340 (1999): 1379.

14 "I was precisely the . . ." The high level of media attention to Reye's syndrome because of its impact on white middle-class rural and suburban children engages many of the same issues that arise in what some sociologists call "missing white women syndrome," which is a drastically elevated level of attention from the media

when young white women disappear. See Cory L. Armstrong, ed., *Media Disparity: A Gender Battleground* (Lanham: Lexington Books, 2013): 21.

15 "In the early 1980s . . ." L. Corey, R. J. Rubin, M. A. Hattwick, G. R. Noble, E. Cassidy, "A Nationwide Outbreak of Reye's Syndrome: Its Epidemiologic Relationship to Influenza B," *American Journal of Medicine* 61 (1976): 615–625. Calvin C. Linnemann, Jr., letter to the editor, *Pediatrics* 68 (1981): 748.

17 "Lately the story of . . ." David Michaels, *Doubt Is Their Product: How Industries Assault on Science Threatens Your Health* (New York: Oxford University Press, 2008): ix–x. A more concise presentation of Michaels's argument can be found in David Michaels and Celeste Monforton, "Manufacturing Uncertainty: Contested Science and the Protection of the Public's Health and Environment," *American Journal of Public Health* 95 (2005): S39–S48.

17 "Clearly, many public health . . ." *Reye's Syndrome: Hearings before the Subcommittee on Natural Resources, Agriculture Research, and Environment of the Committee on Science and Technology, U.S. House of Representatives, Ninety-seventh Congress, second session, September 17 and 29, 1982*, 2122.

19 "Without directly arguing against . . ." Arnold S. Monto, "The Disappearance of Reye's Syndrome—A Public Health Triumph," *Pediatrics* 340 (1999): 1423–1424.

20 "The certainty that eventually . . ." Michael Thaler, personal communication, January 16, 2013.

21 James Orlowski, a Cleveland . . ." James P. Orlowski, Jonathan Gillis, and Henry A. Kilham, "A Catch in the Reye," *Pediatrics* 80 (1987): 638–663.

21 "When I started this . . ." Peter Lurie and Sidney Wolfe, "Aspirin and Reye Syndrome," in *Paradigms for Change: A Public Health Textbook for Medical, Dental, Pharmacy, and Nursing Students* (Washington, DC: Public Citizen Health Research Group, unpublished). The text of "Aspirin and Reye Sundrome" can be found at http://defendingscience.org/sites/default/files/

upload/Lurie_Aspirin.pdf (accessed May 28, 2013). The text that is available online does not attribute the chapter to Lurie and Wolfe, nor does it provide any citation data other than the chapter's title. Citation information was presented in Michaels, *Doubt is Their Product*, xi, 275. I later found Barbara Hinkson Craig, *Courting Change: The Story of the Public Citizen Litigation Group* (Washington, DC: Public Citizen Press, 2004), which contains a chapter on President Ronald Reagan, deregulation, and Public Citizen's efforts to compel the federal government to require labels on aspirin bottles that would warn of its possible relationship to Reye's syndrome.

22 "Lurie and Wolfe's analysis . . ." Lurie and Wolfe, "Aspirin and Reye Syndrome," 1. Lurie and Wolfe's source is E. A. Mortimer, Jr., and M. L. Lepow, "Varicella with Hypoglycemia Possibly Due to Salicylates," 583–590.

22 "For Wolfe, the account . . ." Lurie and Wolfe, "Aspirin and Reye Syndrome," 16.

Chapter One: The Discovery of Reye's Syndrome

25 "It seems that every . . ." R. D. K. Reye, "A Consideration of Certain Subdermal Fibromatous Tumours of Infancy," *Journal of Pathology and Bacteriology* 72 (1956): 149–154. Christina Schnell, Alex Kan, and Kathryn N. North, "'An Artefact Gone Awry': Identification of the First Case of Nemaline Myopathy by Dr. R. D. K. Reye," *Neuromuscular Disorders* 10 (2000): 307–312. Lawrence K. Altman, "Tale of Triumph in Every Bottle," *New York Times* (May 11, 1999): F8. William S. Haubrich, "Reye of Reye's Syndrome," *Gastroenterology* 128 (2005): 1786. Altman, "Tale of Triumph," F8. J. M. Alexander, "Obituary: Ralph Douglas Kenneth Reye," *Australian Pediatric Journal* 14 (1978): 48.

25 "Throughout the 1950s, a . . ." James E. Heubi, *Reye's Syndrome: Because You Need to Know* (Bryan, OH: National Reye's Syndrome Foundation, 2011), 1.

26 “Beginning in 1951 and . . .” James Baral, “Varicella and Herpes Zoster,” *New England Journal of Medicine* 311 (1984): 329. Altman, “Tale of Triumph,” F8. Heubi, *Reye's Syndrome: Because You Need to Know.*

26 “Reye was a notably . . .” Heubi, *Reye's Syndrome.* Ralph Douglas Kenneth Reye, Graeme Morgan, and James Baral, “Encephalopathy and Fatty Degeneration of the Viscera,” *Lancet* (1963): 749–752.

28 “When the seventh patient . . .” Reye, Morgan, and Baral, “Encephalopathy and Fatty Degeneration of the Viscera,” 751, 752.

29 “The doctors were every . . .” Kathryn R. Reeves, “Beware of Reye's Syndrome,” *American Journal of Nursing* 74 (1974): 1621–1622.

30 “Reye and his colleagues' . . .” “Acute Fatty Liver and Coma in Children,” *Lancet* (1963): 772–773. In suggesting similarities between what Reye, Morgan, and Baral had described, the editors of the *Lancet* cited Derrick B. Jelliffe, Gerrit Bras, and Kenneth L. Stuart, “Veno-Occlusive Disease of the Liver,” *Pediatrics* 14 (1954): 334–339. Gerrit Bras and K. R. Hill, “Veno-Occlusive Disease of the Liver: Essential Pathology,” *Lancet* (1956): 161–163. K. R. Hill, C. F. Stephenson, and I. Filshie, “Hepatic Veno-Occlusive Disease: Produced Experimentally in Rats by the Injection of Monocrotaline,” *Lancet* (1958): 623.

30 “In the spring of . . .” Stephen B. Thacker, Andrew L. Dannenberg, and Douglas H. Hamilton, “Epidemic Intelligence Service of the Centers for Disease Control and Prevention: 50 Years of Training and Service in Applied Epidemiology,” *American Journal of Epidemiology* 154 (2001): 985–992. Alexander D. Langmuir, “The Epidemic Intelligence Service of the Center for Disease Control,” *Public Health Reports* 95 (1980): 470–477.

31 “Early in 1962, Johnson . . .” George Magnus Johnson, “Reye's Syndrome—Its American Origins,” *Journal of the National Reye's Syndrome Foundation* 1 (1980): 56–62.

32 “By April, new cases . . .” Johnson, “Reye's Syndrome,” 58.

32 “Johnson found little in . . .” Johnson, “Reye's Syndrome,” 59–60.

33 "Johnson was 'buoyed by . . ." Johnson, "Reye's Syndrome," 60. George Magnus Johnson, Theodore D. Scurletis, and Norma B. Carroll, "A Study of Sixteen Fatal Cases of Encephalitis-Like Disease in North Carolina Children," *North Carolina Medical Journal* 24 (1963): 464–475.

34 "Not being able to . . ." Gilles Lyon, Philip R. Dodge, and R. D. Adams, "The Acute Encephalopathies of Obscure Origin in Infants and Children," *Brain* 84 (1961): 680–708. Johnson, "Reye's Syndrome," 59.

35 "Johnson and his colleagues . . ." Johnson, Scurletis, and Carroll, "Sixteen Fatal Cases of Encephalitis-Like Disease," 471–472.

36 "There does not appear . . ." R. I. K. Elliott, Trevor P. Mann, and F. W. Nash, "Encephalopathy and Fatty Degeneration of the Viscera," *Lancet* (October 26, 1963): 882. W. A . Bourne, "Clinico-Pathological Conference: Liver Disease in Infancy: Held at the Royal Alexandra Hospital for Sick Children," *Postgraduate Medical Journal* 38 (1962): 642–652. Reye and Morgan, "Encephalopathy and Fatty Degeneration of the Viscera," *Lancet* (1963): 1061.

36 "Throughout the mid-1960s . . ."Keitha Corlett, "Encephalopathy and Fatty Degeneration of the Viscera," *Lancet* (November 2, 1963): 937.

37 "Reported cases of encephalitis . . ." H. L. Utian and J. M. Wagner, "Encephalopathy and Fatty Degeneration of the Viscera," *Lancet* (November 9, 1963): 1010. A year later, in 1964, they published a description of three representative cases of what they called "white liver" disease and cited Reye, Morgan, and Baral and several of the reports in the *Lancet* that responded to their 1963 paper. H. L. Utian, J. M. Wagner, and R. J. S. Sichel, "'White-Liver' Disease," *Lancet* (November 14, 1963): 1043. A. F. J. Maloney, "Encephalopathy and Fatty Degeneration of the Viscera," *Lancet* (1963): 1122. D. E. Price, "Encephalopathy and Fatty Degeneration," *Lancet* (1965): 1163. A. W. Blair, W. M. Jamieson, and G. H. Smith, "Complications and Death in Chicken-Pox," *British Medical Journal* 2 (1965): 981–983. Gerald S. Golden and David Duffell, "Encephalopathy and Fatty Change

in the Liver," *Pediatrics* 36 (1965): 67–74 , J. T. Jabbour, Paxton H. Howard, and William E. Jaques, "Encephalopathy and Fatty Degeneration of the Liver and Kidneys, " *Journal of the American Medical Association* 194 (1965): 1245–1247. Martin Randolph, Ramon Kranwinkel, Ronald Johnson, and Nelson A. Gelfman, "Encephalopathy, Hepatitis and Fat Accumulation in Viscera," *American Journal of Diseases in Children* 110 (1965): 95–99. Herbert L. Winograd, "Encephalopathy with Hypoglycemia and Degeneration of the Liver," *Journal of the American Medical Association* 194 (1965): 189–191.

38 "Nonetheless, there was little . . ." A. S. Curry, Helene A. Nathan Guttman, D. E. Price, "A Urinary Pteridine in a Case of Liver Failure," *Lancet* (April 28, 1962): 885–886.

38 "Reye and his coauthors . . ." R. McD. Anderson, "Encephalitis in Childhood: Pathological Aspects," *The Medical Journal of Australia* 50 (1963): 573–575.

38 "Johnson and his colleagues . . ." They cited T. H. Flewett and J. G. Hoult, "Influenzal Encephalopathy and Postinfluenzal Encephalitis," *Lancet* (1958): 11–15. Flewett and Hoult cited V. Dubowitz, "Influenzal Encephalitis," *Lancet* 275 (1960): 61. J. M. Dunbar, W. M. Jamieson, J. H. H. Langlands, G. H. Smith, "Encephalitis and Influenza," *British Medical Journal* 1 (1958): 913–915. R. J. McGill and R. A. Goodbody, "Influenzal Encephalitis," *Lancet* (1958): 320. T. H. Flewettt and J. G. Hoult, "Influenzal Encephalopathy," 11–15. R. N. Compton Smith, "Influenzal Encephalitis," *Lancet* (1958): 217. Cases that appear in the RS literature regarding influenzal encephalitis include R. J. McGill and R. A. Goodbody, "Influenzal Encephalitis," *Lancet* (1958): 320. R. N. Compton Smith, "Influenzal Encephalitis," *Lancet* (1958): 140–141. J. M. Dunbar, W. M. Jamieson, Jean H. M. Langlands, and G. H. Smith, "Encephalitis and Influenza," *British Medical Journal* (1958): 913–915. V. Dubowitz, "Influenzal Encephalitis," *Lancet* (1960): 61.

39 "Johnson and his coauthors . . ." Stuart H. Walker and Yasushi Togo, "Encephalitis Due to Group B, Type 5 Coxsackie Virus," *American Journal of Diseases of Children* 105 (1963): 123–126.

39 "Walker and Togo reported . . ." Gilbert Dalldorf and Grace M. Sickles, "An Unidentified, Filterable Agent Isolated from the Feces of Children with Paralysis," *Science* 108 (1948): 61–62.

Chapter Two: Toxins: The Obvious Cause

42 "In the early 1970s . . ." Samuel L. Katz, "American Academy of Pediatrics Committee on Infectious Diseases Statement on Reye's Syndrome," *Pediatrics* 55 (1975): 139.

42 "While one group of . . ." Allen M. Glasgow, Robert B. Cotton, Kamnual Dhiensiri, and Khon Kaen, "Reye's Syndrome: I. Blood Ammonia and Consideration of the Nonhistolic Diagnosis," *American Journal of Diseases of Children* 124 (1972): 827–833. Frederick J. Samaha, Edward Blau, and John L. Berardinelli, "Reye's Syndrome: Clinical Diagnosis and Treatment with Peritoneal Dialysis," *Pediatrics* 53 (1974): 336–340.

43 "As the diagnostic criteria . . ." Reye, Morgan, and Baral, "Encephalopathy and Fatty Degeneration of the Vicera," 751–752.

43 "The search for a . . ." John F. T. Glasgow and J. A. J. Ferris, "Encephalopathy and Visceral Fatty Infiltration of Probable Toxic Ætiology," *Lancet* 291 (1969): 451–453. M. G. Norman, "Encephalopathy and Fatty Degeneration of the Viscera in Childhood: I. Review of Cases at the Hospital for Sick Children, Toronto (1954–1966)," *Canadian Medical Association Journal* 99 (1968): 522–526.

44 "In the mid-1970s . . ." Emanuel Theodor, Mordechai Ravid, Ronald Jaffe, Bernard E. Cohen, "Fatal Liver Disease of Unknown Origin in Two Adolescent Brothers," *American Journal of Diseases of Children* 128 (1974): 727–730.

45 "In addition to the . . ." Reye, Morgan, and Baral, "Encephalopathy and Fatty Degeneration of the Viscera," 752. Utian and Wagner, "Encephalopathy and Fatty Degeneration of the Viscera," 1010. Utian, Wagner, and Sichel, "'White-Liver' Disease," 1045. Donald G. Barceloux, "Akee Fruit and Jamaican Vomiting Sickness," *Disease-a-Month* June 2009: 318. Barceloux, "Ackee Fruit and Jamaican Vomiting Sickness," 323.

45 "Case reports of people . . ." P. C. Feng, "Hypoglycin from Ackee: A Review," *West Indian Medical Journal* 18 (1969): 238–243. Hassall, K. Reyle, and P. C. Feng, "Hypoglycin A, B: Biologically Active Polypeptides from *Glighia sapida* 173 (1954): 356–357. Kay Tanaka, Kurt J. Isselbacher, Vivian Shih, "Isovaleric and α-Methylbutyric Acidemias Induced by Hypoglycin A: A Mechanism of Jamaican Vomiting Sickness," Science 175 (1972): 69–71.

46 "For several years in . . ." Allen Glasgow and H. Peter Chase, "Production of the Features of Reye's Syndrome in Rats with 4-Pentenoic Acid," *Pediatric Research* 9 (1975): 133–134. M. F. Lowry, "Reye's Syndrome," in E. A. Kean, ed., *Hypoglycin*, edited by E. A. Kean (New York: Academic Press, 1975): 45–54. Kay Tanaka, E. A. Kean, and Barbara Johnson, "Jamaican Vomiting Sickness," *New England Journal of Medicine* 295 (1976): 465.

46 "Other physicians, however, believed . . ." Doris Trauner, William L. Nyhan, and Lawrence Sweetman, "Jamaican Vomiting Sickness and Reye's Syndrome," *New England Journal of Medicine* 295 (1976): 1481. Kay Tanaka, "Reply," *New England Journal of Medicine* 295 (1976): 1481. Ronald A. Chalmers, Alexander M. Lawson, Andrew Whitelaw, and Paul Purkiss, "Twin Siblings with a Reye's Syndrome Associated with Abnormal Organic Aciduria, Hypoglycemia, Diarrhea, and Vomiting with Close Similarities to Jamaican Vomiting Sickness," *Pediatric Research* 14 (1980): 1097. See also R. A. Chalmers, A. M. Lawson, A. Whitelaw, and Paul Purkiss, "Organic Acids in Reye's Like Syndrome: Similarities with Jamaican Vomiting Sickness," *Lancet* 8022 (1977): 1156–1157.

48 "In 1966, the same . . ." D. M. O. Becroft, "Syndrome of Encephalopathy and Fatty Degeneration of the Viscera in New Zealand Children," *British Medical Journal* 2 (1966): 135–140.

48 "The condition of the . . ." Becroft, "Syndrome of Encephalopathy and Fatty Degeneration of Viscera," 139.

49 "Aflatoxins had been first . . ." "Aflatoxin," *Lancet* (May 16, 1964): 1090. P. G. Tulpule, T. V. Madhavan, and C. Gopalan, "Effect of Feeding Aflatoxin to Young Monkeys," *Lancet* (May

2, 1964): 962–963. Becroft, "Syndrome of Encephalopathy and Fatty Degeneration of Viscera," 139. Robin Barr, Irving H. J. Glass, and Gurbachan S. Chawla, "Reye's Syndrome: A Massive Fatty Metamorphosis of the Liver with Acute Encephalopathy," *Canadian Medical Association Journal* 98 (1968): 1043.

49 "By far the most . . ." C. H. Bourgeois, N. Keschamras, D. S. Comer, S. Harikul, H. Evans, L. Olson, T. Smith, M. Beck, "Udorn Encephalopathy: Fatal Cerebral Edema and Fatty Degeneration of the Viscera in Thai Children," *Journal of the Medical Associaiton of Thailand* 52 (1969), 553–555, 558.

50 "As had Reye and . . ." Bourgeois, Keschamras, Comer, Harikul, Evans, Olson, Smith, Beck, "Udorn Encephalopathy," 561.

50 "Over the next several . . ." Ronald Shank, Dennis O. Johnsen, Prayot Tanticharoenyos, William L. Wooding, and Curtis H. Bourgeois, "Acute Toxicity of Aflatoxin B1 in the Macaque Monkey," *Toxicology and Applied Pharmacology* 20 (1971): 227–231. Curtis H. Bourgeois, Ronald Shank, Richard Grossman, Dennis O. Johnsen, William L. Wooding, and Pramukh Chandavimol, "Acute Aflatoxin B1 Toxicity in the Macaque and Its Similarities to Reye's Syndrome," *Laboratory Investigation* 24 (1971): 206–215.

51 "Having already shown with . . ." Lloyd C. Olson, Curtis H. Bourgeois, Robert B. Cotton, Supha Harikul, Richard Grossman, and Thomas J. Smith, "Encephalopathy and Fatty Degeneration of the Viscera in Northeastern Thailand: Clinical Syndrome and Epidemiology," *Pediatrics* 47 (1971): 707–716.

52 "Near the end of . . ." Curtis Bourgeois, Lloyd Olson, Dhira Comer, Hilary Evans, Niyom Keschamras, Robert Cotton, Richard Grossman, and Thomas Smith, "Encephalopathy and Fatty Degeneration of the Viscera: A Clinicopathologic Analysis of 40 Cases," *American Journal of Clinical Pathology* 56 (1971): 558–571.

53 "In retrospect, it might . . ." An example of later authorities who presented the SEATO researchers' findings as informative only of children in Thailand was M. Michael Thaler, "Reye's Syndrome:

Cause-and-Effect Relationships," in Samuel R. Berenberg, ed., *Liver Diseases in Infancy and Childhood* (New York: Springer, 1976): 72–83.

53 "The SEATO researchers themselves . . ." Bourgeois, Shank, Grossman, Johnsen, Wooding, and Chandavimol, "Acute Aflatoxin B1 Toxicity in the Macaque," 215. Olson, Bourgeois, Cotton, Harikul, Grossman, and Smith, "Encephalopathy and Fatty Degeneration of the Viscera," 715. R. C. Shank, C. H. Bourgeois, N. Keschamras, and P. Chandavimol, "Aflatoxins in Autopsy Specimens from Thai Children with an Acute Disease of Unknown Aetiology," *Food and Cosmetics Toxicology* 9 (1971), 506. The group was similarly restrained in concluding that their findings only illuminated the cause of a select group of Thai children's ailments in Bourgeois, Olson, Comer, Evans, Keschamras, Cotton, Grossman, and Smith, "Encephalopathy and Fatty Degeneration of the Viscera," 570.

53 "I think the aflatoxins . . ." Olson, Bourgeois, Cotton, Harikut, Grossman, and Smith, "Encephalopathy and Fatty Degeneration of the Viscera," 712.

54 "Throughout the 1970s, the . . ." D. M. O. Becroft and D. R. Webster, "Aflatoxins and Reye's Disease," *British Medical Journal* 4 (1972): 117. I. Dvorackova, J. Zilkova, and J. Cerman, "Aflatoxin and the Encephalitic Syndrome Associated with Fatty Organs," *Ceskoslovenska Gastroenterologie Vyziva* 9-27 (1973): 551–552. I. Dvorackova, J. Zilkova, and J. Brodsky, J. Cerman, "Aflatoxin and Liver Damage with Encephalopathy," *Sb Ved Pr Lek Fak Karlovy Univerzity Hradci Kralove* 15 (1972): 521–524. Enrique Chaves-Carballo, Ralph D. Ellefson, Manuel R. Gomez, "An Aflatoxin in the Liver of a Patient with Reye-Johnson Syndrome," *Mayo Clinic Proceedings* 51 (1976): 48–50. Gwendolyn R. Hogan, Nell J. Ryan, A. Wallace Hayes, "Aflatoxin and Reye's Syndrome," *Lancet* (1978): 561.

54 "In 1979, the University . . ." Peter R. Huttenlocher and Doris A. Trauner, "Reye's Syndrome in Infancy," *Pediatrics* 62 (1978): 84–90. Nell J. Ryan, Gwendolyn R. Hogan, A. Wallace Hayes, Peter Unger, and Mohamed Y. Siraj, "Aflatoxin B1: Its Role in the Etiology of Reye's Syndrome," *Pediatrics* 64 (1979): 71–75.

55 "The mounting circumstantial evidence . . ." C. J. Mann, "Observational Research Methods," *Emergency Medicine Journal* 20 (2003): 54–60.

55 "Any question of whether . . ." David B. Nelson, Renate Kimbrough, Philip S. Landrigan, A. Wallace Hayes, George C. Yange, and Jeannette Benanides, "Aflatoxin and Reye's Syndrome: A Case Control Study," *Pediatrics* 66 (1980): 865–869

CHAPTER THREE: The Deadly Mist

57 "In 1962, a year . . ." Rachel Carson, *Silent Spring* (New York: Houghton Mifflin, 1962). Eliza Griswold, "How 'Silent Spring' Ignited the Environmental Movement," *New York Times Magazine* (September 21, 2012).

58 "In the early 1970s . . ." "NRSF 35th Annual Meeting: Dr John Crocker, SAB Member," http://www.youtube.com/watch?v=sDjRDpptQIA (accessed June 2, 2014).

58 "The insecticides that Crocker . . ." J. R. Blais, "Trends in the Frequency, Extent, and Severity of Spruce Budworm Outbreaks in Eastern Canada," *Canadian Journal of Forest Research* 13 (1983): 539–547. T. Royama, W. E. MacKinnon, E. G. Kettela, N. E. Carter, and L. K. Hartling, "Analysis of Spruce Budworm Outbreak Cycles in New Brunswick, Canada, Since 1952," *Ecology* 86 (2005): 1222.

59 "To limit the impact . . ." "TBM Avengers & Forest Protection Limited—New Brunswick, Canada: Information Archive," www.http://forestprotectiontbmavengers.wordpress.com/about/ (accessed February 25, 2013).

59 "Given growing concerns over . . ." Carson, *Silent Spring*, 121–122. J. J. Fettes and C. H. Buckner, "Historical Sketch of the Philosophy of Spruce Budworm Control in Canada," in *Proceedings of a*

Symposium on the Spruce Budworm, November 11–14, 1974, Alexandria, Virginia, United States Department of Agriculture, Forest Service, Miscellaneous Publication No. 1327: 58.

60 "DDT was used on . . ."W. M. Ciesla, "*Historical and Present Approach to Spruce Budworm Control in the United States*," in *Proceedings of a Symposium on the Spruce Budworm, November 11–14, 1974, Alexandria, Virginia*, United States Department of Agriculture, Forest Service, Miscellaneous Publication No. 1327: p,. 53. Fettes and Buckner, "Historical Sketch of the Philosophy of Spruce Budworm Control in Canada," 58–59. M. F. Mitchell and J. R. Roberts, "A Case Study of the Use of Fenitrothion in New Brunswick: The Evolution of an Ordered Approach to Ecological Monitoring," in Patrick J. Sheehand, Donald R. Miller, George, C. Butler, and Philippe Bourdeau, eds., *Effects of Pollutants at the Ecosystem Level* (Hoboken: John Wiley & Sons, 1984): 377–402.

60 "By the mid-1970s . . ." Russell Hunt, "Biological Warfare in New Brunswick," *Ottawa Journal Weekend Magazine* (August 7, 1976): 11–15. Mark J. McLaughlin, "Green Shoots: Aerial Insecticide Spraying the Growth of Environmental Consciousness in New Brunswick, 1952–1973," *Acadiensis* 40 (2011): 4–5.

61 "From the start, scientists . . ." C. J. Kerswill and P. F. Elson, "Preliminary Observations on Effects of 1954 DDT Spraying on Atlantic Salmon," *Progress Reports, Atlantic Coast Stations, Fisheries Research Board, Canada* 62 (1955): 17–24. Ott Hicks, "DDT Kills Salmon, Spraying Operations Puts Salmon Crop in Jeopardy," *Rod and Gun in Canada* 57 (August 1955): 5, 17. McClaughlin, "Green Shoots," 11, 12.

62 "In January 1972, a . . ." Hunt, "Biological Warfare in New Brunswick": 11–15.

62 "Timmy Keddy was one . . ." Hunt, "Biological Warfare in New Brunswick": 11–15.

62 "By the early 1970s . . ." M. Friend and D. O. Trainer, "Polychlorinated Biphenyl: Interaction with Duck Hepatitis Virus," *Science* 170 (1970): 1314–1316. "NRSF 35th Annual Meeting: Dr John Crocker, SAB Member," http://www.youtube.com/watch?v=sDjRDpptQIA (accessed June 2, 2014)

63 "Despite the perceived threat . . ." Crocker and his colleagues cited work that had been done with young ducks and published three years earlier: Friend and Trainer, "Polychlorinated Biphenyl." John F. S. Crocker, Kenneth R. Rozee, R. L. Ozere, Sharon C. Digout, and O. Hutzinger, "Insecticide and Viral Interaction as a Cause of Fatty Visceral Changes and Encephalopathy in the Mouse," *Lancet* (July 6, 1974): 22–24.

63 "Crocker's goal of identifying . . ." Crocker, Rozee, Ozere, Digout, and Hutzinger, "Insecticide and Viral Interaction as a Cause of Fatty Visceral Changes," 22, 23.

64 "Even though the results . . ." Alan Miller, *Environmental Problem Solving: Psychosocial Barriers to Adaptive Change,* New York: Springer, 1999): 107. "NRSF 35th Annual Meeting: Dr John Crocker, SAB Member," http://www.youtube.com/watch?v=sDjRDpptQIA (accessed June 2, 2014).

64 "Upon closer scrutiny and . . ." J. F. S. Crocker et al., "Lethal Interaction of Ubiquitous Insecticide Carriers with Virus.," *Science* 192, no. 4246 (June 25, 1976): 1351–1353.

65 "In March 1976, several . . ." Miller, "The Role of Citizen Scientist in Nature Resource Decision-Making," 50–51. H. Versteeg, "The Spruce Budworm Programme and the Perception of Risk in New Brunswick," in *Pesticide Policy: The Environmental Perspective* (Ottawa: Friends of the Earth, 1984). Quoted in Miller, "The Role of Citizen Scientist in Nature Resource Decision-Making," 51–52. "Rare Children's Disease Tied To Solvents Used in Pesticides," *New York Times* (April 10, 1976). "Rare Children's Disease Tied To Solvents Used in Pesticides," *New York Times* (April 10, 1976). "NRSF 35th Annual Meeting: Dr John Crocker, SAB Member," http://www.youtube.com/watch?v=sDjRDpptQIA (accessed June

2, 2014). Alan Miller, "The Role of Citizen Scientist in Nature Resource Decision-Making: Lessons from the Spruce Budworm Problem in Canada," *The Environmentalist* 13 (1993): 51.

65 "Unlike Nova Scotia, where . . ." Tom Spears, "From Farm Boy to NRC Chief," *Ottawa Citizen*, March 9, 2013. W. G. Schneider, G. C. Butler, J. S. Campbell, J. S. Migicovsky, B. B. Morley, and M. G. Forest, *Forest Spray Programme and Reye's Syndrome: Report of the Panel Convened by the Government of New Brunswick* (Fredericton: Government of New Brunswick, 1976).

66 "As the expert panel's . . ." "Parents Plea for End to Budworm Spraying," *Ottawa Journal* (April 5, 1976).

66 "Given the inconclusive findings . . ." See for example Michaels, *Doubt is Their Product* and Mark A. Largent, *Vaccine: The Debate in Modern America* (Baltimore: Johns Hopkins University Press, 2012).

67 "In the face of . . ." Margaret Carrol, "Canadian Woman Warns of Aerial Spraying," *Bangor Daily News* (August 19, 1977). Miller, *Environmental Problem Solving,* 106. Miller cited "Public 'Mistrusts' Forest Spraying," *Daily Gleaner* (February 19, 1969).

79 "Over the summer of . . ." "Ontario Will Spray Against the Budworm," *Ottawa Journal* (May 25, 1976). Hunt, "Biological Warfare in New Brunswick": 15. "Spraying Budworm Prevented 'Forest Becoming Tinderbox,'" *Ottawa Journal* (September 1, 1976).

68 "New Brunswick's 1976 spraying . . ." Allan Chambers, "Chemical Warfare on Worms—What are the Dangers?" *Ottawa Journal* (May 15, 1976): 8. Peter Meerburg, "To Spray or Not to Spray Is Question 'Bugging' NS," *Ottawa Journal* (December 9, 1976): 7. Hunt, "Biological Warfare in New Brunswick:" 11–15.

68 "Hunt's article elicited a . . ." Carol Dumont, letter to the editor, *Ottawa Journal Weekend Magazine* (September 18, 1976): 3. L. A. Adams, letter to the editor, *Ottawa Journal's Weekend Magazine* (September 26, 1976): 8.

69 "The lack of definitive . . ." Meerberg, "To Spray or Not to Spray is Question 'Bugging' NS," 7. Marlene Simmons, "More Study Urged for Spruce Budworm Spray," (December 29, 1976).

69 "A court case involving aerial . . ." Allan Chambers, "Budworm Debate Moved into Court," *Ottawa Journal* (December 27, 1977). George W. Schuyler, "Chemical Warfare in Canada," *New York Times* (May 23, 1979): A27.

70 "In April 1977, as . . ." J. D. Pollack, J. H. Hughes, V. V. Hamparian, and D. Burech, "The Interaction of Chemicals and Viruses and Their Role in Reye's Syndrome," *Chemosphere* 7 (1978): 551–563.

70 "A year later, Crocker . . ." Pollack, Hughes, Hamparian, and Burech, "The Interaction of Chemicals and Viruses and Their Role in Reye's Syndrome," 551–563. John F. S. Crocker, editorial, *Chemosphere* 7 (1978): v. The articles in the issue were Pollack, Hughes, Hamparian, and Burech, "Interaction of Chemicals and Viruses and Their Role in Reye's Syndrome," 551–563. P. C. Bagnell, John F. S. Crocker, and R. L. Ozere, "Reye's Syndrome in Canada's Maritime Provinces," *Chemosphere* 7 (1978): 565–571. Spencer H. S. Lee, Kenneth R. Rozee, Stephen H. Safe, and John F. S. Crocker, "The Properties of Emulsifiers that Enhance the Replication of Viruses in Cell Cultures," *Chemosphere* 7 (1978): 573–589. D. J. Ecobichon, John F. S. Crocker, "Depression of Blood Cholinesterases as a Marker of Spray Exposure," *Chemosphere* 7 (1978): 591–596. John F. S Crocker, Sharon Digout, P. Bagnell, Spencer H. S. Lee, Kenneth R. Rozee, and S. Safe, "Viral Interaction with Pesticide Emulsifiers in Vivo," *Chemosphere* 7 (1989): 597–606. J. Sparling, B. Chittim, B. S. Clegg, S. Safe, and John F. S. Crocker, "The Tissue Distribution and Clarence of Aerotex 3470, an Aromatic Hydrocarbon Solvent," *Chemosphere* 7 (1978): 607–614. J. M McLeod and J. McNeil, "Fenitrothion: Apparent Long-Term Effects on Larvae of a Sawfly," *Chemosphere* 7 (1978): 615–619.

70 "Resistance to Canadian provinces' . . ." David Agnew, "Spray Scheme Protest Grows," *Ottawa Journal* (June 10, 1978): 8. "Boy's Death Linked to Budworm Spray," *Ottawa Journal* (April 27, 1979): 8. "Television Schedule," *Ottawa Journal* (June 15, 1979):

23. Mike Strobel, "Spray Wars! Are the Risks Worth the Results?" *Ottawa Journal* (September 17, 1979): 27. Carolyn Belardo, "Despite Controversy, State Presses Spraying Program," *New York Times* (December 7, 1980): NJ2.

71 "Throughout the late 1970s . . ." Kenneth R. Rozee, Spencer H. S. Lee, John F. S. Crocker, and Stephen H. Safe, "Enhanced Virus Replication in Mammalian Cells Exposed to Commercial Emulsifiers," *Applied and Environment Microbiology* 35 (1978): 297–300.

72 "As the aspirin hypothesis . . ." S. H. S. Lee, M. Laltoo, J. F. S. Crocker, and Kenneth R. Rozee, "Emulsifiers that Enhance Susceptibility to Virus Infection: Increased Virus Penetration and Reduced Interferon Response," *Applied and Environmental Microbiology* 40 (1980): 878–793. Kenneth R. Rozee, S. H. S. Lee, John F. S. Crocker, Sharon C. Digout, E. Arcinue, "Is a Compromised Interferon Response an Etiologic Factor in Reye's Syndrome?" *Canadian Medical Association Journal* 136 (1983): 798–802. John F. S. Crocker, S. H. S. Lee, J. A. Love, D. A. Malatjalian, K. W. Renton, Kenneth R. Rozee, and M. G. Murphy, "Surfactant-Potentiated Increases in Intracranial Pressure in a Mouse Model of Reye's Syndrome," *Environmental Neurology* 111 (1991): 95–97. John F. S. Crocker, Sharon C. Digout, Spencer H. Lee, Kenneth R. Rozee, Ken Renton, Chris A. Field, Philip Acott, Mary G. Murphy, "Effects of Antipyretics on Mortality Due to Influenza B Virus in a Mouse Model of Reye's Syndrome," *Clinical and Investigative Medicine* 21 (1998): 192–202. "NRSF 35th Annual Meeting: Dr John Crocker, SAB Member," http://www.youtube.com/watch?v=sDjRDpptQIA (accessed June 2, 2014). See also M. G. Murphy, Sharon C. Digout, and John F. S. Crocker, "Animal Models for Reye's Syndrome," in A. Boulton, G. Baker, and R. Butterworth, eds., *Neuromethods, Volume 22: Animal Models of Neurological Disease, II* (New York: Humana Press, Inc., 1992): 223–257.

72 "In the early 1980s . . ." Bert Deveaux, "The Poison Mist: A Special Investigation into New Brunswick's Forest Spray Programme," Canadian Broadcasting Corporation (January 3, 1982). See also

Michael S. Kramer, "Kids Versus Trees: Reye's Syndrome and Spraying for Spruce Budworm in New Brunswick," *Journal of Clinical Epidemiology* 62 (2009): 579.

73 "As public concdern about . . ." Michael S. Kramer, "Kids Versus Trees: Reye's Syndrome and Spraying for Spruce Budworm in New Brunswick," *Journal of Clinical Epidemiology* 62 (2009): 579. Kenneth R. Rozee, S. H. S. Lee, John F. S. Crocker, Sharon Digout, and E. Arcinue, "Is a Compromised Interferon Response an Etiologic Factor in Reye's Syndrome?" *Canadian Medical Journal* 126 (1982): 802. Robert B. Wood, Jr., and Gregory F. Bogdan, "Reye's Syndrome and Spruce Budworm Insecticide Spraying in Maine, 1978–1982," *American Journal of Epidemiology* 124 (1986): 671. Deveaux, "The Poison Mist." Rozee's statements were also presented in "Halifax Scientist Links Children's Disease to Chemicals Used on Spruce Budworm," *Montreal Gazette*, January 4, 1982.

74 "'Science' is often popularly . . ." For examples of the "science says . . ." approach, see Russell A. Barkley and Kevin R. Murphy, *ADHD in Adults: What the Science Says* (New York: Guilford Press, 2010); Jamie Whyte, "Science Says So, Suckers!" *Wall Street Journal* (August 14, 1013); and Liz Neporent, "Mean Girl Behavior is the Norm, Science Says," ABC News Blog http://abcnews.go.com/blogs/health/2013/10/30/mean-girl-behavior-is-the-norm-science-says/ (accessed October 31, 2013). The United States Centers for Disease Control funds, in part, a series of research briefs titled *Science Says*. The National Campaign to Prevent Teen and Unplanned Pregnancy, "Science Says," http://www.thenationalcampaign.org/resources/sciencesays.aspx (accessed October 31, 2013).

74 "Health and environmental issues . . ." McLaughlin, "Green Shoots," 12. Kerswill and Elson, "Preliminary Observations on Effects of 1954 DDT Spraying on Atlantic Salmon," 17–24. Hicks, "DDT Kills Salmon, Spraying Operations Puts Salmon Crop in Jeopardy," 5, 17. Hunt, "Biological Warfare in New Brunswick," 13. Allan Chambers, "Budworm Debate Moved into Court," *Ottawa Journal* (December 27, 1977).

75 "On of the ways . . ." Michael S. Kramer, "Kids Versus Trees: Reye's Syndrome and Spraying for Spruce Budworm in New Brunswick," *Journal of Clinical Epidemiology* 62 (2009): 579.

75 "The task force flew . . ." In Ohio, the published rate was 1.04 cases per 100,000 persons, and in Michigan it was estimated that Reye's syndrome appeared in between 30.8 and 57.8 cases of Influenza B. See John Z. Sullivan-Bolyai, James S. Marks, Deane Johnson, David B. Nelson, Frank Holtzhauer, Frank Bright, Taylor Kramer, and Thomas J. Halpin, "Reye Syndrome in Ohio, 1973-1977," *American Journal of Epidemiology* 112 (1980): 629–638 and Lawrence Corey, Robert, J. Rubin, Theodore R. Thompson, Gary R. Noble, Edward Cassidy, Michael A. W. Hattwick, Michael B. Gregg, and Donald Eddins, " Influenza B-Associated Reye's Syndrome Incidence in Michigan and Potential for Prevention," *Journal of Infectious Diseases* 135 (1977): 398–407. Kramer, "Kids Versus Trees," 580. The report they produced was Walter O. Spitzer, Michael A. Hattwick, Eugene Hurwitz, Michael Kramer, Lawrence Kupper, R. P. Bryce Larke, J. Dennis Pollack, Ronald Shank, Patrick Seliske, "Report of the New Brunswick Task Force on the Environment and Reye's Syndrome." *Clinical Investigative Medicine* 5 (1982): 203e14.

76 "Shortly after Spitzer's New . . ." Robert B. Wood, Jr., and Gregory F. Bogdan, "Reye's Syndrome and Spruce Budworm Insecticide Spraying in Maine, 1978-1982," *American Journal of Epidemiology* 124 (1986): 677.

Chapter Four: The Front Line in the Battle against Reye's Syndrome

79 "The authors of the . . ." "Encephalopathy and Fatty Infiltration of Viscera in Children," *Lancet* (1969): 473–475.

79 "While there was considerable . . ." See for example Emanuel Theodor, Mordechai Ravid, Ronald Jaffe, and Bernard Cohen, "Fatal Liver Disease of Unknown Origin in Two Adolescent Brothers," *American Journal of Diseases of Children* 128 (1974): 727–730 and Rickey Wilson, Jenelle Miller Harry Greene, Robert Rankin, Lawrence Lumeng, David Gordon, David Nelson, and

Gary Noble, "Reye's Syndrome in Three Siblings: Association with Type A Influenza Infection," *American Journal of Diseases of Children* 134 (1980): 1032–1034.

81 "In contrast to the . . ." "Reye's Syndrome: Dr. William Schubert—1976," http://www.youtube.com/watch?v=Fg5pUJdCbRk

82 "Stage I: vomiting, lethargy . . ." Frederick H. Lovejoy, Jr., Arnold L. Smith, Michael J. Bresnan, James N. Wood, David I. Victor, and Patricia C. Adams, "Clinical Staging in Reye Syndrome," *American Journal of Diseases of Children* 128 (1974): 36–41.

83 "Reye and his colleagues . . ." Reye, Morgan, and Baral, "Encephalopathy and Fatty Degeneration of the Viscera," 750–751.

84 "The SEATO researchers in . . ." Bourgeois, Keschamras, Comer, Harikul, Evans, Olson, Smith, Beck, "Udorn Encephalopathy," 558.

85 "As physicians developed therapies . . ." James P. Orlwoski, Usasma, A. Hanhan, and Mariano R. Fiallo, "Is Aspirin a Cause of Reye's Syndrome? A Case Against," *Drug Safety* 25 (2002): 230.

86 "While some physicians focused . . ." Henry Nadler, "Therapeutic Delirium in Reye's Syndrome," *Pediatrics* 54 (1974): 265–266.

86 "Peter R. Huttenlocher, a . . ." John Easton, "Peter Huttenlocher, Pediatric Neurologist," *UChicago News* (August 19, 2013).

86 "Huttenlocher's firsts contribution to . . ." Peter R. Huttenlocher, Allen D. Schwartz, and Gerald Klatskin, "Reye's Syndrome: Ammonia Intoxication as a Possible Factor in the Encephalopathy," *Pediatrics* 43 (1969): 443–454.

87 "As a diagnostic tool . . ." Huttenlocher, Schwartz, and Klatskin, "Reye's Syndrome," 451.

87 "Huttenlocher and his colleagues . . ." Huttenlocher et al cited G. S. Golden and D. Dufell, "Encephalopathy and Fatty Change in the Liver and Kidneys," *Pediatrics* 36 (1965): 67; Utian, Wagner, and Sichel, "'White Liver' Disease," 1043; Dvorackova, Vortel, and Hroch, "Ecephalitic Syndrome with Fatty Degeneration of the

Liver," 1247; and R. A. Joske, D. D. Keall, P. J. Leak, N. F. Stanley, M. N. I. Walters, "Hepatitis-Encephalitis in Humans with Reovirus Infection," *Archives of Internal Medicine* 113 (1964): 811.

88 "Whatever therapies emerged, it . . ." Huttenlocher, Schwartz, and Klatskin, "Reye's Syndrome," 451.

88 "In the 1960s, as . . ." Charles Trey, Derrick G. Burns, and Stuart J. Saunders, "Treatment of Hepatic Coma by Exchange Blood Transfusion," *New England Journal of Medicine* 274 (1966): 473–481.

88 "The first physicians to . . ." Charles Trey and A. Tink, "Exchange Transfusion in Hepatic Coma: Report of Case," *Medical Journal of Australia* 1 (1958): 40–42. Trey, Burns, Saunders, "Treatment of Hepatic Coma by Exchange Blood Transfusion," 473. Robert L. Berger, Rodney M. Liversage, Thomas C. Chalmers, James H. Graham, David M. McGoldrich, and Frederick Stohlman, Jr. "Exchange Transfusion in the Treatment of Fulminating Hepatitis," *New England Journal of Medicine* 274 (1966): 497–499. J. M Burnell, J. K. Dawborn, R. B. Epstien, R. A. Gutman, G. E. Leinboach, E. D. Thomas, and W. Volwiler, "Acute Heaptic Coma Treated by Cross-Circulation or Exchange Transfusion," *New England Journal of Medicine* 276 (1967): 935–943.

89 "Citing the research on . . ." A. P. Hart, "Familial Icterus Gravis of the New-Born and Its Treatment," *Canadian Medical Association Journal* 15 (1925): 1008–1011.

89 "Of the ten children . . ." Huttenlocher, Schwartz, and Klatskin, "Reye's Syndrome," 453.

90 "The protocol that Huttenlocher . . ." Peter R. Huttenlocher, "Reye's Syndrome: Relation of Outcome to Therapy," *Journal of Pediatrics* 80 (1972): 845–850.

91 "The 1976 film on . . ." "In Memoriam: William Kenneth Schubert," http://www.cincinnatichildrens.org/news/release/2012/schubert-memoriam/ (accessed December 26, 2013).

91 "Schubert appeared in the . . ." "Reye's Syndrome: Dr. William Schubert—1976," http://www.youtube.com/watch?v=Fg5pUJdCbRk (accessed December 26, 2013).

92 "Schubert, Partin, and their . . ." Jacqueline S. Partin, Cynthia C. Daugherty, A. James McAdams, John C. Partin, and William K. Schubert, "A Comparison of Liver Ultrastructure in Salicylate Intoxication and Reye's Syndrome," *Hepatology* 4 (1984): 687–690. "Reye's Syndrome: Dr. William Schubert—1976," http://www.youtube.com/watch?v=Fg5pUJdCbRk (accessed December 26, 2013).

92 "In 1975, Schubert and . . ." William K. Schubert, Robert C. Bobo, John C. Partin, and Jacqueline S. Partin, "Reye's Syndrome," *Disease-a-Month* (1975).

92 "The physicians at Cincinnati . . ." Schubert, Bobo, Partin, and Partin, "Reye's Syndrome," 22. Robert C. Bobo, William K. Schubert, John C. Partin, and Jacqueline S. Partin, "Reye Syndrome: Treatment by Exchange Transfusion with Special Reference to the 1974 Epidemic in Cincinnati, Ohio," *Journal of Pediatrics* 87 (1975): 881–886.

93 "Even more dramatic than . . ." Azmy R. Boutros, Shahpour Esfandiari, James P. Orlowski, and Jonathan, S. Smith, "Reye's Syndrome: A Predictably Curable Disease," *Pediatric Clinics of North America* 27 (1980): 539–552. A. Bengerovskii, I. V. Sukhodolo, V. S. Chuchlain, A. G. Arbuzov, M. B. Chervyakova, Yu Yu Mel'nik, E. I. Grishina, and A. S. Saratikov, "Therapeutic Efficacy of Legalon and Lokhein with Respect to Experimental Reye's Syndrome," *Pharmaceutical Chemistry Journal* 34 (2000): 165–167. R. C. McWilliam and J. B. P. Stephenson, "Life-Threatening Intracranial Hypertension in Reye's Syndrome Treated with Intravenous Thiopentone," *European Journal of Pediatrics* 144 (1985): 383–384.

93 "When drugs alone could . . ." Timothy C. Frewen, David B. Swedlow, Mehernoor Watcha, Russell C. Raphaely, Rodolfo I. Godinez, Mark S. Heiser, Robert G. Kettrick, and Derek A. Bruce, "Outcome in Severe Reye Syndrome with Early Pentobarbital

Coma and Hypothermia," *Journal of Pediatrics* 100 (1982): 663–665. Kevin Drum, "Drug Coma Slows Child's Rare Disease," *Los Angeles Times* (February 6, 1981): A1. Doris A. Trauner, "What Is the Best Treatment for Reye's Syndrome," *Archives of Neurology*, 43 (1986): 729.

94 "Perhaps the most dramatic . . ." Barr, Glass, and Chawla, "Reye's Syndrome," 1038–1044. Schubert, Bobo, Partin, and Partin, "Reye's Syndrome," 25–26. Partin, Partin, Schubert, and McLaurin, "Brain Ultrastructure in Reye's Syndrome," 426–427. "Brain Ultrastructure in Reye's Syndrome," 427.

95 "Given their obvious personal . . ." Partin, Partin, Schubert, and McLaurin, "Brain Ultrastructure in Reye's Syndrome," 427.

96 "Throughout the 1970s and . . ." *National Reye's Syndrome Foundation, 1974-2009* (Bryan, OH: National Reye's Syndrome Foundation, Inc.): 2009.

Chapter Five: The Aspirin Hypothesis

98 "Throughout the 1960s and . . ." Calvin C. Linnemann, Jr., "letter to the editor," *Pediatrics* 68 (1981): 748.

98 "Aspirin's history stretches back . . ." J. G. Mahdi, A. J. Mahdi, A. J. Mahdi, and I. D. Bowen, "The Historical Analysis of Aspirin Discovery, Its Relation to the Willow Tree and Antiproliferative and Anticancer Potential," *Cell Proliferation* 39 (2006): 147.

99 "From the 1850s through . . ." Mahdi, Mahdi, Mahdi, and Bowen, "Historical Analysis of Aspirin Discovery," 149.

99 "For decades, credit for . . ." Walter Sneader, "The Discovery of Aspirin: A Reappraisal," *British Medical Journal* 321 (2000): 1591.

100 "Bayer had quickly recognized . . ." Eleanor Berman, "Review of *Salicylates: An International Symposium*," *Journal of the American Medical Association* (1964): 1162.

100 "While it was hard . . ." E. A. Mortimer and Martha Lipson Lepow, "Varicella with Hypoglycemia Possibly Due to Salicylates," *American Journal of Diseases of Children* 103 (1962): 586, 589–590.

101 "Most of the early . . ." Utian, Wagner, and Sichel, "'White-Liver' Disease," 1043.

102 "The first to suggest . . ." H. McC. Giles, "Encephalopathy and Fatty Degeneration of the Viscera," *Lancet* (1965): 1075.

102 "Given that ultimately aspirin . . ." Lyon, Dodge, and Adams, "Acute Encephalopathies of Obscure Origin in Infants and Children," 702–703.

102 "In 1965, four physicians . . ." George Limbeck, Rogelio Ruvalcaba, Ellis Samols, and Vincent C. Kelley, "Salicylates and Hypoglycemia," *American Journal of Diseases of Children* 109 (1965): 165–167. Reye, "Encephalopathy and Fatty Degeneration of the Viscera," 752.

103 "Given the results of . . ." Martin Gross and Leon A. Greenberg, *The Salicylates: A Critical Bibliographic Review* (New Haven: Hillhouse Press, 1948): 108–109. Dwight J. Ingle, "Effect of Aspirin Upon Glycosuria of the Partially Depancreatized Rat," *Proceedings of the Society of Experimental Biology and Medicine* 75 (1950): 673–674. M. J. H. Smith, B. W. Meade, and J. Bornstein, "The Effect of Salicylate on Glycosuria, Blood Glucose and Liver Glycogen of the Alloxan-Diabetic Rat," *Biochemical Journal* 51 (1952): 18–20. M. J. H. Smith, "The Effect of Salicylate on the Glycosuria and Hyperglycaemia Induced by Cortisone in the Normal Rat," *Biochemical Journal* 52 (1952): 649–652. Cecilia Lutwak-Mann, "The Effect of Salicylate and Cinchophen on Enzymes and Metabolic Processes," *Biomedical Journal* 36 (1942): 10–12.

104 "By the mid-1960s . . ." Randall Baselt, *Disposition of Toxic Drugs and Chemicals in Man*, 8th Edition (Foster City: Biomedical Publications, 2008): 22–25. M. G. Norman, "Encephalopathy and Fatty Degeneration of the Viscera in Childhood: I. Review of Cases at The Hospital for Sick Children, Toronto (1954-1966)," *Canadian Medical Association Journal* 99 (1968): 522–526.

104 "An authoritative rejection of . . ." Thomas H. Glick, William H. Likosky, Lawrence P. Levitt, Harold Mellin, and David W. Reynolds, "Reye's Syndrome: An Epidemiologic Approach," *Pediatrics* 46 (1970): 371–377.

105 "But other government agencies . . ." "Reye's Syndrome: Etiology Uncertain But Avoid Antiemetics in Children," *FDA Drug Bulletin* 6 (1976): 40–41. John Z. Sullivan-Boyai and Lawrence Corey, "Epidemiology of Reye Syndrome," *Epidemiologic Reviews* 3 (1981): 1–26.

105 "Researchers and physicians working . . ." Mark Pendergrast, *Inside the Outbreaks: The Elite Medical Detectives of the Epidemic Intelligence Service* (New York: Houghton Mifflin Harcourt, 2010): 118. Thomas H. Glick, William H. Likosky, Lawrence P. Levitt, Harold Mellin, and David W. Reynolds, "Reye's Syndrome: An Epidemiologic Approach," *Pediatrics* 46 (1970): 371–377. Glick, Likosky, Levitt, Mellin, Reynolds, "Reye's Syndrome," 376.

106 "In the latter half . . ." Lawrence Corey, Robert J. Rubin, Dennis Bregman, and Michael B. Gregg, "Diagnostic Criteria for Influenza B-Associated Reye's Syndrome: Clinical vs. Pathologic Criteria," *Pediatrics* 60 (1977): 706.

107 "The first strong epidemiological . . ." Karen Starko, George Ray, Lee B. Dominguez, Warren L. Strongberg, and Dora F. Woodall, "Reye's Syndrome and Salicylate Use," *Pediatrics* 66 (1980): 859–864. Personal correspondence with Karen Starko, February 18, 2014.

107 "In the spring of 1979 . . ." "NRSF 35th Annual Meeting: Lawrence Schonberger, M.D., M.P.H., CDC—YouTube," https://www.youtube.com/watch?v=izr2V17l4FQ (accessed March 18, 2014).

107 "Starko had not been . . ." Personal correspondence with Karen Starko, February 18, 2014. Pendergrast, *Inside the Outbreaks,* 190.

108 "Starko found it was . . ." "NRSF 35th Annual Meeting: Lawrence Schonberger, M.D., M.P.H., CDC—YouTube," https://www.youtube.com/watch?v=izr2V17l4FQ (accessed March 18, 2014). Personal correspondence with Karen Starko, February 18, 2014.

108 "In the paper in *Pediatrics* . . ." Starko, Ray, Dominguez, Strongberg, and Woodall, "Reye's Syndrome and Salicylate Use," 863.

109 "Starko and her colleagues . . ." Starko, Ray, Dominguez, Strongberg, and Woodall, "Reye's Syndrome and Salicylate Use," 863.

109 "It took the better . . ." William M. Young, "Doubts Relationship of Salicylate and Reye's Syndrome," *Pediatrics* 68 (1981): 466–467. Joseph H. Clark and Joseph F. Fitzgerald, "Doubts Relationship of Salicylate and Reye's Syndrome," *Pediatrics* 68 (1981): 467. D. Grant Gall and Geoffrey Barker, "Doubts Relationship of Salicylate and Reye's Syndrome," *Pediatrics* 68 (1981): 467–468.

110 "Starko and C. George . . ." Karen M. Starko and C. George Ray, "Doubts Relationship of Salicylate and Reye's Syndrome," *Pediatrics* 68 (1981): 468. Starko and Ray quoted Thomas Sydenham's "Concerning Peruvian Bark and the Intermitting Fever."

111 "The same year that . . ." E. Chaves-Carballo, "Epidemiology of Reye Syndrome," *Advances in Neurology* 19 (1978): 231–248. John Z. Sullivan-Bolyai, James S. Marks, Deane Johnson, David B. Nelson, Frank Holtzhauer, Frank Bright, Taylor Kramer, and Thomas J. Halpin, "Reye Syndrome in Ohio, 1973-1977," *American Journal of Epidemiology* 112 (1980): 629–638.

111 "There was nothing in . . ." "Reye's Syndrome—Ohio, Michigan," *Morbidity and Mortality Weekly Report* 29 (1980): 532–539.

112 "The editors of the . . ." "Reye's Syndrome—Ohio, Michigan," 537–539.

113 "Michigan experienced some of . . ." Gene Schroeder, "Reye's Syndrome Victim's Mother Tells Sad Story," *News-Palladium* (March 8, 1974): 12. "Michigan Reports Most Reye's Cases," *News-Pallidium* (March 8, 1974): 12. "Critical Health Problems Reporting Act," Michigan Act 312 (1978).

114 "Empowered by the state's . . ." Ronald J. Waldman, William N. Hall, Harry McGee, George Van Amburg, "Aspirin as a Risk Factor in Reye's Syndrome," *Journal of the American Medical Association* 247 (1982): 3089–3094.

114 "In their initial study . . ." Waldman, Hall, McGee, Van Amburg, 3090–3091.

115 "Like me, Harry McGee . . ." Author's interview with Harry McGee, February 20, 2014.

115 "The goal of the . . ." Author's interview with Harry McGee, February 20, 2014.

116 "After reports emerged from . . ." Iver Peterson, "Children's Disease Jolts a Small Town in Michigan," *New York Times* (February 24, 1980).

117 "News that officials might . . ." "Studies Warn Parents about Link of Aspirin to Childhood Disease," *New York Times* (November 8, 1981). Sandy Rovner, "Health Talk: Reye's Syndrome," *Washington Post* (January 23, 1981): B5. "Doctors Alert for Reye's Syndrome: Illness, Possibly Aspirin-Linked, Affects Young People," *Lost Angeles Times* (February 8, 1981): 6. Committee on Infectious Diseases, American Academy of Pediatrics, "Reye's Syndrome and Aspirin," *Indian Journal of Pediatrics* 48 (1981): 455.

117 "The initial reports all . . ." "Reye Syndrome—Ohio, Michigan," 538–539. "Studies Warn Parents about Link of Aspirin to Childhood Disease." Committee on Infectious Diseases, American Academy of Pediatrics, "Reye's Syndrome and Aspirin," 455.

119 "Aspirin consumption alone, however . . ." Karen Starko, "A Few Questions and Answers on Reye's Syndrome," The Science Blogs Book Club http://scienceblogs.com/bookclub/2010/07/07/a-few-questions-and-answers-on/ (accessed December 29, 2013). Paul F. Pinsky, Eugene S. Hurwitz, Lawrence B. Schonberger, and Walter J. Gunn, "Reye's Syndrome and Aspirin: Evidence for a Dose-Response Effect," *Journal of the American Medical Association* 260 (1988): 857–861.

119 "Late in 1980, the . . ." Quoted in *Public Citizen Health Research Group v. Commission, Food & Drug Administration, and Aspirin Foundation of America, Inc.*, 740 F.2d 21, 238 US App., DC 271. Cristine Russell, "Children with Chicken Pox, Flue Shouldn't Use Aspirin, US Says," *Washington Post* (February 12, 1982): A3.

Vincent A. Fulginiti, Philip A. Brunell, James D. Cherry, Walton L. Ector, Anne A. Gershon, Samuel P. Gotoff, Walter T. Hughes, Jr., Edward A. Mortimer, Jr., and Georges Peter, "Aspirin and Reye Syndrome," *Pediatrics* 1982 (69): 810–812. "Academy of Pediatrics Warns of Aspirin Risk," *Washington Post* (May 20, 1982: A18. Michael DeCourcy Hinds, "Aspirin Linked to Children's Disease," *New York Times* (April 28, 1982). Michael DeCourcy Hinds, "Warning Issued on Giving Aspirin to Children," *New York Times* (June 5, 1982).

Chapter Six: The Aspirin Industry Responds

122 "Almost as soon as . . ." Michaels and Monforton, "Manufacturing Uncertainty," S39.

122 "Throughout the summer and . . ." Hinds, "Warning Issued on Giving Aspirin to Children."

123 "In April 1982, just . . ." "Announcement: Aspirin Foundation," *Diseases of the Colon & Rectum* 25 (1982): 250.

123 "Joseph White, the first . . ." Charles R. Babcock, "Aspirin Makers Vow Fight Over Warning," *Washington Post* (June 6, 1982): A4. "Aspirin Link to Disease Challenged," *New York Times* (June 9, 1982). For examples of publicity about White's claims, see Sharon Cohen, "Aspirin Industry Vows Warning Label Fight," *Free Lance-Star*, Fredericksburg, VA (June 6, 1982) and "Campaign Directed at Alerting Parents on Aspirin-Syndrome Link," *Galveston Daily News*, Galveston, TX (September 21, 1982).

124 "The clearest articulation of . . ." Author's interview with Harry McGee, February 20, 2014. RS Working Group, "Reye Syndrome and Salicylates: A Spurious Association," *Pediatrics* 70 (1982): 158–160.

124 "The Aspirin Foundation of . . ." The Aspirin Foundation, "Aspirin and Reye's Syndrome," http://www.aspirin-foundation.com/suitability/backgrounder.html (accessed March 21, 2014).

125 "Sometime in 1982, a . . ." Lurie and Wolfe, "Aspirin and Reye Syndrome," 11–12.

125 "A third pro-aspirin industry . . ." "Emergency Reye's Syndrome Prevention Act of 1985," *Hearings Before the Subcommittee on Health and the Environment of the Committee on Energy and Commerce, House of Representatives, Ninety-Ninth Congress,* March 15, 1985 (Washington, DC: US Government Printing Office, 1985): 310.

125 "The aspirin industry-funded . . ." RS Working Group, "Reye Syndrome and Salicylates," 160.

126 "In September 1982, as . . ." *Reye's Syndrome: Hearings before the Subcommittee on Natural Resources, Agriculture Research, and Environment of the Committee on Science and Technology, U.S. House of Representatives, Ninety-seventh Congress, second session, September 17 and 29, 1982*, 1.

127 "The hearing opened with . . ." *Reye's Syndrome: Hearings before the Subcommittee on Natural Resources, Agriculture Research, and Environment of the Committee on Science and Technology, U.S. House of Representatives, Ninety-seventh Congress, second session, September 17 and 29, 1982*, 10–11.

128 "Scheuer politely interrupted Johnson's . . ." *Reye's Syndrome: Hearings before the Subcommittee on Natural Resources, Agriculture Research, and Environment of the Committee on Science and Technology, U.S. House of Representatives, Ninety seventh Congress, second session, September 17 and 29, 1982*, 11–12.

128 "For Johnson, the question . . ." The discussion in *Pediatrics* to which Johnson referred in his testimony was Brunell, Cherry, Ector, Gershon, Gotoff, Hughes, Mortimer, and Peter, "Special Report: Aspirin and Reye's Syndrome," 810–812 and Wilson and Brown, "Reye Syndrome and Aspirin Use," 822–825. In his testimony, Johnson made reference to "Wilson" in the context of descripting parents' errors in accurately recalling the medications they had given their children. Given Johnson's earlier reference to the June issue of *Pediatrics*, it appears that he is referring to Wilson and Brown, "Reye's Syndrome and Aspirin Use," 822–825. *Reye's Syndrome: Hearings before the Subcommittee on Natural Resources,*

Agriculture Research, and Environment of the Committee on Science and Technology, U.S. House of Representatives, Ninety-seventh Congress, second session, September 17 and 29, 1982, 12–13.

129 "Johnson's claim that his . . ." *Reye's Syndrome: Hearings before the Subcommittee on Natural Resources, Agriculture Research, and Environment of the Committee on Science and Technology, U.S. House of Representatives, Ninety-seventh Congress, second session, September 17 and 29, 1982*, 13–14.

129 "Scheuer followed Johnson's prepared . . ." *Reye's Syndrome: Hearings before the Subcommittee on Natural Resources, Agriculture Research, and Environment of the Committee on Science and Technology, U.S. House of Representatives, Ninety-seventh Congress, second session, September 17 and 29, 1982*, 21–22.

130 "After Johnson's testimony concluded . . ." *Reye's Syndrome: Hearings before the Subcommittee on Natural Resources, Agriculture Research, and Environment of the Committee on Science and Technology, U.S. House of Representatives, Ninety-seventh Congress, second session, September 17 and 29, 1982*, 25–26, 31.

130 "Unlike Johnson, Eichenwald had . . ." *Reye's Syndrome: Hearings before the Subcommittee on Natural Resources, Agriculture Research, and Environment of the Committee on Science and Technology, U.S. House of Representatives, Ninety-seventh Congress, second session, September 17 and 29, 1982*, 26.

131 "Eichenwald had access to . . ." In the transcript of the hearing, Robert Hoekelman's name is misspelled as Robert Heckelman, Philip Lanzkowsky's name is misspelled as Phillip Manskoski, and Henry Nadler's name is misspelled as Henry Madler. *Reye's Syndrome: Hearings before the Subcommittee on Natural Resources, Agriculture Research, and Environment of the Committee on Science and Technology, U.S. House of Representatives, Ninety-seventh Congress, second session, September 17 and 29, 1982*, 26. "Drug Firms Aren't Likely to See Big Aspirin Profit," *Lawrence Journal-World* (January 27, 1988). *Reye's Syndrome: Hearings before the Subcommittee on Natural Resources, Agriculture Research, and*

Environment of the Committee on Science and Technology, U.S. House of Representatives, Ninety-seventh Congress, second session, September 17 and 29, 1982, 26–27, 35, 56.

131 "In the question-and- . . ." *Reye's Syndrome: Hearings before the Subcommittee on Natural Resources, Agriculture Research, and Environment of the Committee on Science and Technology, U.S. House of Representatives, Ninety-seventh Congress, second session, September 17 and 29, 1982*, 35, 37.

132 "The testimony offered by . . ." *Reye's Syndrome: Hearings before the Subcommittee on Natural Resources, Agriculture Research, and Environment of the Committee on Science and Technology, U.S. House of Representatives, Ninety-seventh Congress, second session, September 17 and 29, 1982*, 39.

132 "Paul Hinson, the executive . . ." In the transcript, Hinson was incorrectly identified in the hearing transcripts as the Executive Director of the National Reye's Syndrome Foundation, which was and still is based in Dayton, Ohio. In fact, Hinson was the Executive Director of the American Reye's Syndrome Foundation, which is no longer in existence and was based in Denver, Colorado. *Reye's Syndrome: Hearings before the Subcommittee on Natural Resources, Agriculture Research, and Environment of the Committee on Science and Technology, U.S. House of Representatives, Ninety-seventh Congress, second session, September 17 and 29, 1982*, 48.

133 "The testimonies critical of . . ." *Reye's Syndrome: Hearings before the Subcommittee on Natural Resources, Agriculture Research, and Environment of the Committee on Science and Technology, U.S. House of Representatives, Ninety-seventh Congress, second session, September 17 and 29, 1982*, 57, 63.

133 "Other than the first . . ." For information on Bach, see Brit Allan Storey, "Oral History Interviews: Maryanne C. Bach," http://www.usbr.gov/history/OralHistories/BACH,%20MARYANNE%20MASTER%20I,%20CIT,%20NF,%20S,%20OC,%20AE,%20HI,%20HC,%20FN,%20SC,%20INSERTS,%20CREATE.%20MAR,%20BACH%20EDITS,%20SoD%20AND%20INSERTS%20

REMOVED.pdf (accessed May 14, 2013). *Reye's Syndrome: Hearings before the Subcommittee on Natural Resources, Agriculture Research, and Environment of the Committee on Science and Technology, U.S. House of Representatives, Ninety-seventh Congress, second session, September 17 and 29, 1982*, 66–67.

134 "The first witness to . . ." *Reye's Syndrome: Hearings before the Subcommittee on Natural Resources, Agriculture Research, and Environment of the Committee on Science and Technology, U.S. House of Representatives, Ninety-seventh Congress, second session, September 17 and 29, 1982*, 68.

134 "Unlike the previous witnesses . . ." *Reye's Syndrome: Hearings before the Subcommittee on Natural Resources, Agriculture Research, and Environment of the Committee on Science and Technology, U.S. House of Representatives, Ninety-seventh Congress, second session, September 17 and 29, 1982*, 70–71.

134 "The next witness, Reule . . ." *Reye's Syndrome: Hearings before the Subcommittee on Natural Resources, Agriculture Research, and Environment of the Committee on Science and Technology, U.S. House of Representatives, Ninety-seventh Congress, second session, September 17 and 29, 1982*, 71, 72.

135 "Stallones reported that there . . ." *Reye's Syndrome: Hearings before the Subcommittee on Natural Resources, Agriculture Research, and Environment of the Committee on Science and Technology, U.S. House of Representatives, Ninety-seventh Congress, second session, September 17 and 29, 1982*, 73.

136 "As a result of . . ." *Reye's Syndrome: Hearings before the Subcommittee on Natural Resources, Agriculture Research, and Environment of the Committee on Science and Technology, U.S. House of Representatives, Ninety-seventh Congress, second session, September 17 and 29, 1982*, 73.

136 "While a subtle change . . ." *Reye's Syndrome: Hearings before the Subcommittee on Natural Resources, Agriculture Research, and Environment of the Committee on Science and Technology, U.S. House of Representatives, Ninety-seventh Congress, second session, September 17 and 29, 1982*, 78.

137 "Scheuer opened the second . . ." *Reye's Syndrome: Hearings before the Subcommittee on Natural Resources, Agriculture Research, and Environment of the Committee on Science and Technology, U.S. House of Representatives, Ninety-seventh Congress, second session, September 17 and 29, 1982*, 81–82, 86–87. Eugene S. Hurwitz, Michael J. Barrett, Dennis Bregman, Walter J. Gunn, Lawrence B. Schonberger, William R. Fairweather, Joseph S. Drage, John R. LaMontagne, Richard A. Kaslow, D. Bruce Burlington, Gerald V. Quinnan, Robert A. Parker, Kem Phillips, Paul Pinsky, Delbert Dayton, and Walter R. Dowdle, "Public Health Service Study on Reye's Syndrome and Medications: A Report on the Pilot Phase," *New England Journal of Medicine* 313 (1985): 849–857. Eugene S. Hurwitz, Michael J. Barrett, Dennis Bregman, Walter J. Gunn, Paul Pinsky, Lawrence B. Schonberger, Joseph S. Drage, Richard A. Kaslow, D. Bruce Burlington, Gerald V. Quinnan, John R. LaMontagne, William R. Fairweather, Delbert Dayton, and Walter R. Dowdle, "Public Health Service Study of Reye's Syndrome and Medications: Report of the Main Study," *Journal of the American Medical Association* 257 (1987): 1905-1912.

138 "Brandt, fully aware that . . ." "Reye Syndrome—Ohio, Michigan," *Morbidity and Mortality Weekly Report* (November 7, 1980): 532–539. "National Surveillance for Reye Syndrome, 1981: Update, Reye Syndrome and Salicylate Usage," *Morbidity and Mortality Weekly Report* (February 12, 1982): 53–56, 61. *Reye's Syndrome: Hearings before the Subcommittee on Natural Resources, Agriculture Research, and Environment of the Committee on Science and Technology, U.S. House of Representatives, Ninety-seventh Congress, second session, September 17 and 29, 1982*, 82–84.

138 "Brandt explained that, based . . ." *Reye's Syndrome: Hearings before the Subcommittee on Natural Resources, Agriculture Research, and Environment of the Committee on Science and Technology, U.S. House of Representatives, Ninety-seventh Congress, second session, September 17 and 29, 1982*, 85.

139 "In the question-and- . . ." *Reye's Syndrome: Hearings before the Subcommittee on Natural Resources, Agriculture Research, and Environment of the Committee on Science and Technology, U.S. House of Representatives, Ninety-seventh Congress, second session, September 17 and 29, 1982*, 87.

139 "Shacknai had in hand . . ." *Reye's Syndrome: Hearings before the Subcommittee on Natural Resources, Agriculture Research, and Environment of the Committee on Science and Technology, U.S. House of Representatives, Ninety-seventh Congress, second session, September 17 and 29, 1982*, 88–89.

140 "For the next several . . ." *Reye's Syndrome: Hearings before the Subcommittee on Natural Resources, Agriculture Research, and Environment of the Committee on Science and Technology, U.S. House of Representatives, Ninety-seventh Congress, second session, September 17 and 29, 1982*, 91–92.

140 "Scheuer and Shacknai responded . . ." *Reye's Syndrome: Hearings before the Subcommittee on Natural Resources, Agriculture Research, and Environment of the Committee on Science and Technology, U.S. House of Representatives, Ninety-seventh Congress, second session, September 17 and 29, 1982*, 94.

141 "It would seem at . . ." *Reye's Syndrome: Hearings before the Subcommittee on Natural Resources, Agriculture Research, and Environment of the Committee on Science and Technology, U.S. House of Representatives, Ninety-seventh Congress, second session, September 17 and 29, 1982*, 95.

141 "Scheuer and Shacknai spent . . ." *Reye's Syndrome: Hearings before the Subcommittee on Natural Resources, Agriculture Research, and Environment of the Committee on Science and Technology, U.S. House of Representatives, Ninety-seventh Congress, second session, September 17 and 29, 1982*, 108.

142 "Orlowski was an excellent . . ." *Reye's Syndrome: Hearings before the Subcommittee on Natural Resources, Agriculture Research, and Environment of the Committee on Science and Technology, U.S. House of Representatives, Ninety-seventh Congress, second session, September 17 and 29, 1982*, 114–115.

143 "Scheuer's decision to call . . ." Jennifer Lee, "James H. Scheuer, 13-Term New York Congressman, Is Dead at 85," *New York Times* (August 31, 2005).

143 "According to Scheuer's opening . . ." *Reye's Syndrome: Hearings before the Subcommittee on Natural Resources, Agriculture Research, and Environment of the Committee on Science and Technology, U.S. House of Representatives, Ninety-seventh Congress, second session, September 17 and 29, 1982*, 1–2.

144 "Shacknai was obviously central . . ." *Reye's Syndrome: Hearings before the Subcommittee on Natural Resources, Agriculture Research, and Environment of the Committee on Science and Technology, U.S. House of Representatives, Ninety-seventh Congress, second session, September 17 and 29, 1982*, 80. "Schering Set to Add Key," *New York Times* (March 8, 1986). Deadly New Accusations: A Murder Mystery," Dr. Phil Show (September 21, 2012) http://drphil.com/shows/show/1874 (accessed May 14, 2013). For information on the deaths of Max Shacknai and Rebecca Mawii Zahau, see Elizabeth Vargas, Jessica Hopper, and Christina Caron, "Mansion Deaths: Jonah Shacknai Wants Review of Investigation," ABC News (September 20, 2011) http://abcnews.go.com/US/mansion-deaths-jonah-shacknai-files-letter-investigation-rebecca/story?id=14562097#.UZJx_JVhNcA (accessed May 14, 2013), "Max Shacknai, Son of Millionaire Jonah Shacknai, Was Likely Murdered: Report," Huffingtonpost.com (August 8, 2012) http://www.huffingtonpost.com/2012/08/08/max-shacknai-murdered-jonah-shacknai-report_n_1757919.html (accessed May 14, 2013) and "Jonah Shacknai," radaronline.com http://radaronline.com/category/tags/jonah-shacknai/ (accessed May 14, 2013).

Chapter Seven: The Rise of Labels and the Fall of Reye's

146 "However, just as the . . ." Quoted in Kathleen Browne Ittig, "The Consumer Movement in the United States," *Bridgewater Review* 2 (1983): 11.

147 "Perhaps even more influential . . ." William Kleinknecht, *The Man Who Sold the World: Ronald Reagan and the Betrayal of Main Street America* (New York: Nation Books, 2010): 111. Chris Mooney, *The Republican War on Science* (New York: Basic Books, 2006): 104–105.

147 "Tozzi had come to . . ." "Profile—OMB's Jim Joseph Tozzi," *The Environmental Forum* (May, 1982): 11.

148 "Known to his staff as . . ." Peter Behr, "If There's a New Rule, Jim Tozzi Has Read It," *Washington Post* (July 10, 1981): A21. "Regulatory Officials Shift," *Washington Post* (May 16, 1983). Naomi Oreskes and Erik M. Conway, *Merchants of Doubt: How a Handful of Scientists Obscured the Truth on Issues from Tobacco Smoke to Global Warming* (New York: Bloomsbury Press, 2010): 148.

148 "On the eve of . . ." Tim Miller, "The O.M.B. Writes a Prescription," *The Nation* (March 21, 1984): 383. Behr, "If There's a New Rule, Jim Tozzi Has Read It," A21. Larry Doyle, "Threat of Suits Delayed Warning Process," *Los Angeles Times* (May 31, 1987): 1.

149 "For a public statement . . ." Jonah Shacknai, "Aspirin and the Danger of Childhood Disease," *Wall Street Journal* (October 15, 1982): 34. Miller, "O.M.B. Writes a Prescription," 384.

149 "Armed with Shacknai's op-ed . . ." Gregg Easterbrook, "Ideas Move Nations: How Conservative Think Tanks Have Helped to Transform the Terms of Political Debate," *Atlantic* (January 1986). Miller, "O.M.B. Writes a Prescription," 384.

150 "As representatives from the . . ." Doyle, "Threat of Suits Delayed Warning Process." Miller, "O.M.B. Writes a Prescription," 384. Russell, "HHS Wants More Study on Aspirin Rule," A3.

150 "Gioven the AAP's apparent . . ." Miller, "O.M.B. Writes a Prescription," 384. "US Seeks New Study on Reye's Syndrome," *The New York Times* (November 19, 1982). Cristine Russell, "HHS Wants More Study on Aspirin Rule," *Washington Post* (November 19, 1982): A3.

151 "Nonetheless, Schweiker announced that . . ." Russell, "HHS Wants More Study on Aspirin Rule," A3.

151 "In the end, aspirin . . ." Miller, "O.M.B. Writes a Prescription," 385.

152 "The consumer movement in . . ." Upton Sinclair, *The Jungle* New York: Doubleday, 1906). Pure Food and Drug Act, *United States Statutes at Large* (59th Cong., Session I, Chapter 3915, 768–772; cited as 34 US Stats. 768). Milton Handler, "The Control of False Advertising Under the Wheeler-Lea Act," *Law and Contemporary Problems* (1939): 91. Pure Food and Drug Act, Pub. No 717, 75th Cong. 3d Sess. (June 25, 1938) c. 675, 52 Stat. 1040 (1938), 21 US.C.A., C. 9 (Supp. 1938).

152 "Throughout the first half . . ." Public Citizen, "About Us," http://www.citizen.org/about/ (accessed May 28, 2013).

153 "Public Citizen's efforts to . . ." Sidney Wolfe, "Medical Monitors: Public Health Advocacy Exposes Threats, Educates Consumers," *Public Health News*, http://www.citizen.org/documents/publichealth.pdf (last accessed March 18, 2014). Andis Robeznieks, "Wolfe Resigns as Director of Public Citizen Health," *Modern Healthcare* (June 3, 2013) http://www.modernhealthcare.com/article/20130603/MODERNPHYSICIAN/306039975# (accessed March 18, 2014).

153 "After recounting the studies . . ." United State Court of Appeals, District of Columbia Circuit, *Public Citizen Health Research Group* v. *Commission, Food and Drug Administration, and Aspirin Foundation of America* 740 F.2d 21 238 US App. D.C. 271, No. 83-1302, Argued December 7, 1983, Decided July 27, 1984.

154 "The court approached the . . ."*Nader* v. *FCC*, 520 F.2d 182, 207 (D.C. Cir. 1975). *Public Citizen Health Research Group* v. *Auchter*, supra, 702 F.2d at 1157.

154 "HRG's request to the . . ." "Judicial Review—Actions Reviewable," *Duke Law Journal* 115 (1972): 276–292.

155 "Despite recognizing that 'the . . ." "Advance Notice of Proposed Rulemaking," supra, 47 *Federal Register* 57886, JA 449.

157 "The report from the . . ." Eugene S. Hurwitz, Michael J. Barrett, Dennis Bregman, Walter J. Gunn, Lawrence B. Schonberger, William R. Fairweather, Joseph S. Drage, John R. LaMontagne, Richard A. Kaslow, D. Bruce Burlington, Gerald V. Quinnan, Robert A. Parker, Kem Phillips, Paul Pinsky, Delbert Dayton, and Walter R. Dowdle, "Public Health Service Study on Reye's Syndrome and Medications: Report of the Pilot Phase," *New England Journal of Medicine* 313 (1985): 849–857.

158 "Generic Components of Medications . . ." Hurwitz, Barrett, Bregman, Gunn, Schonberger, Fairweather, Drage, LaMontagne, Kaslow, Burlington, Quinnan, Parker, Phillips, Pinsky, Dayton, and Dowdle, "Public Health Service Study on Reye's Syndrome and Medications," 849–857.

158 "The main study appeared . . ." Eugene S. Hurwitz, Michael Barrett, Dennis Bregman, Walter J. Gunn, Paul Pinsky, Lawrence B. Schonberger, Joseph S. Drage, Richard A. Kalsow, Bruce Burlington, Gerald V. Quinan, John R. LaMontagne, William R. Fairweather, Delbert Dayton, and Walter R. Dowdle, "Public Health Service Study of Reye's Syndrome and Medication: Report of the Main Study," *Journal of the American Medical Association* 257 (1987): 1911.

159 "Generic Components of Medications . . ." Hurwitz, Barrett, Bregman, Gunn, Pinsky, Schonberger, Drage, Kalsow, Burlington, Quinan, LaMontagne, Fairweather, Dayton, and Dowdle, "Public Health Service Study of Reye's Syndrome and Medication: 1911.

160 "Annual Number of Reported . . ." Eugene Hurwitz, David B. Nelson Cornelia Davis, David Morens, and Lawrence B. Schonberger, "National Surveillance for Reye Syndrome: A Five-Year Review," Pediatrics 70 (1982): 895–900. "Reye Syndrome Surveillance—United States, 1986," *Morbidity and Mortality Weekly Report* 36 (October 23, 1987): 689–691. "Reye Syndrome Surveillance—United States, 1987 and 1988," *Morbidity and Mortality Weekly Report* 38 (May 12, 1989): 325–327. "Reye Syndrome Surveillance—United States, 1989," *Morbidity and Mortality Weekly Report* 40 (February 8, 1991): 88–90. Eyelyn Zamula, "Reye's Syndrome: The Decline of a Disease," FDA

Publication No. 94-1172, June 1994. Kevin M. Sullivan, Ermias D. Belay, Randy E. Durbin, David A. Foster, and Dale F. Nordenberg, "Epidemiology of Reye's Syndrome, United States, 1991–1994: Comparison of CDC Surveillance and Hospital Admission Data," *Neuroepidemiology* 19 (2000): 228–344.

160 "There also emerged evidence . . ." Patrick L. Remington, Diane Rowley, Harry McGee, William N. Hall, and Arnold S. Monto, "Decreasing Trends in Reye Syndrome and Aspirin Use in Michigan, 1979 to 1984," *Pediatrics* 776 (1986): 93–98. Janet B. Arrowsmith, Dianne L. Kennedy, Joel N. Kuritsky, and Gerald A. Faich, "National Patterns of Aspirin Use and Reye Syndrome Reporting, United States, 1980 to 1985," *Pediatrics* 79 (19870: 858–863.

161 "The final report of the . . ." Devra Lee Davis and Patricia Buffler, "Reduction of Deaths after Drug Labeling for Risk of Reye's Syndrome," *Lancet* 340 (1992): 1042. "Delay on Aspirin Warning Label Cost Children's Lives, Study Says," *New York Times* (October 23, 1992).

Chapter Eight: Labels, At Last

162 "In January 1985, a . . ." Myron Struck, "Aspirin Warning Labels," *Washington Post* (March 1, 1985): A17. "Mrs. Heckler Urging Syndrome Warning as an Aspirin Label," *New York Times* (January 10, 1985). "Mrs. Heckler Urging Syndrome Warning as an Aspirin Label," *New York Times* (January 10, 1985). "Aspirin Maker to Put Warning On its Labels," *Washington Post* (January 11, 1985): A5. "Makers of Aspirin Endorse Warning," *New York Times* (January 12, 1985). "Warning to Go on Aspirin Labels," *New York Times* (January 24, 1985).

162 "By the mid-1980s . . ." Fred Beard, "An Historical Analysis of the US Advertising Industry's Self-Regulation of Comparative Advertising," *Proceedings of the 15th Biennial Conference on Historical Analysis and Research in Marketing*, May 19–22, 2011. http://faculty.quinnipiac.edu/charm/CHARM%20proceedings/CHARM%20article%20archive%20pdf%20format/Volume%2015%202011/An%20Historical%20analysis%20of%20US%20

Advertising%20industry.pdf (accessed June 12, 2013). Steven Fox, *The Mirror Makers: A History of American Advertising and Its Creators* (New York: Vintage Books, 1984): 126.

163 "In the 1960s, when . . ." Lisa L. Sharma, Stephen P. Teret, and Kelly D. Brownell, "The Food Industry and Self-Regulation: Standards to Promote Success and to Avoid Public Health Failures," *American Journal of Public Health* 100 (2010): 240.

164 "The adoption of self-enforced . . ." Sharma, Teret, Brownell, "The Food Industry and Self-Regulation," 245.

165 "Just as the PMRC . . ." "Reye's Syndrome Warning Bill Emphasizing 'Strong Association' with Aspirin Introduced Feb. 28: Voluntary Warning Program is 'Failing,' Rep. Waxman Says," *The Pink Sheet* 47 (March 4, 1985).

166 "Henry Waxman, the liberal . . ." "Drug Price Competition and Patent Term Restoration Act," Public Law 98-417. United States House of Representatives Committee on Government Reform, Minority Staff Special Investigations Division, "The Content of Federally Funded Abstinence-Only Education Programs," Prepared for Representative Henry A. Waxman, December 2004.

166 "Waxman opened his subcommittee's . . ." "Emergency Reye's Syndrome Prevention Act of 1985," *Hearings Before the Subcommittee on Health and the Environment of the Committee on Energy and Commerce, House of Representatives, Ninety-Ninth Congress*, March 15, 1985 (Washington, DC: US Government Printing Office, 1985): 276. "Voluntary Aspirin Warnings' Success Disputed: Rep. Waxman Outlines Shortfalls at Reye's Syndrome Hearing" *Washington Post* (March 16, 1985): A9. A video of a portion of this hearing is available at "1985 Emergency Reye's Syndrome Act—Part I," http://www.youtube.com/watch?v=kgkD0NWmwBM

167 "Waxman's short opening statement . . ." "Emergency Reye's Syndrome Prevention Act of 1985," 281–282, 283.

167 "Waxman thanked Metzenbaum and . . ." "Emergency Reye's Syndrome Prevention Act of 1985," 284.

168 "Given the striking difference . . ." "Emergency Reye's Syndrome Prevention Act of 1985," 281, 284.

169 "The first group of . . ." "Emergency Reye's Syndrome Prevention Act of 1985," 285–6.

169 "John and Terri Freudenberger . . ." "Emergency Reye's Syndrome Prevention Act of 1985," 287.

169 "Freudenberger testified that authorities . . ." National Reye's Syndrome Foundation, "NRSF 35th Annual Meeting: Lawrence Schonberger," (http://www.youtube.com/watch?v=izr2V17l4FQ). "Emergency Reye's Syndrome Prevention Act of 1985," 286–87.

170 "The last two statements . . ." "Emergency Reye's Syndrome Prevention Act of 1985," 306–308.

171 "The second surprise that . . ." "Emergency Reye's Syndrome Prevention Act of 1985," 315–316.

171 "The second group of . . ." "Emergency Reye's Syndrome Prevention Act of 1985," 318.

171 "Wolfe was followed by . . ." "Emergency Reye's Syndrome Prevention Act of 1985," 319–20, 322.

172 "By the end of . . ." "Emergency Reye's Syndrome Prevention Act of 1985," 309, 321. Starko and Ray, "Doubts Relationship of Salicylate and Reye's Syndrome,"468.

172 "Both of the first . . ." "Emergency Reye's Syndrome Prevention Act of 1985," 318.

173 "Frank Young, the commissioner . . ." "Emergency Reye's Syndrome Prevention Act of 1985," 326.

173 "In the question-and- . . ." "Emergency Reye's Syndrome Prevention Act of 1985," 361, 413.

173 "The last set of . . ." "Emergency Reye's Syndrome Prevention Act of 1985," 276, 463, 489.

174 "Despite White's claims, researchers . . ." Richard S. K. Young, Dennis Torretti, Robert H. Williams, Donald Hendriksen, and Michael Woods, "Reye's Syndrome Associated with Long-Term

Aspirin Therapy," *Journal of the American Medical Association* 251 (1984): 754–756. Patrick L. Remington, Charles L. Shabino, Harry McGee, Greg Preston, Ashock P. Sarniak, and William N. Hall, "Reye Syndrome and Juvenile Rheumatoid Arthritis in Michigan," *American Journal of Diseases of Children* 139 (1985): 870–872. See also J. Roger Hollister, "Aspirin in Juvenile Rheumatoid Arthritis," *American Journal of Diseases of Children* 139 (1985): 866–867.

175 "James Cope took an . . ." "Consumer Healthcare Products Association, "About CHPA," http://www.chpa-info.org/aboutchpa/about_chpa.aspx (accessed June 17, 2013). The Proprietary Association was founded in 1881, changed its name to the Nonprescription Drug Manufacturers Association in 1989 and to the Consumer Healthcare Products Association in 1999. "Emergency Reye's Syndrome Prevention Act of 1985," 518–520.

175 "The third and final . . ." "Dispute on Aspirin Continues," *The Palm Beach Post* (November 25, 1982): A14. "Emergency Reye's Syndrome Prevention Act of 1985," 540.

175 "The subcommittee hearing concluded . . ." "Emergency Reye's Syndrome Prevention Act of 1985," 641–643.

176 "The record of the . . ." "Emergency Reye's Syndrome Prevention Act of 1985," 704–707.

176 "By the fall of . . ." "FDA Proposes Label on Aspirin Warning of Link to Disease," *Wall Street Journal* (September 21, 1982): 24. Marlene Cimons, "Stronger Warning Label on Aspirin Urged: House Subcommittee Wants Link to Reye's Syndrome Mentioned," *Los Angeles Times* (October 24, 1985).

177 "The new label, with . . ." Marlene Cimons, "'Agreement in Principle' Reached on Aspirin Label Telling of Reye's Syndrome," *Los Angeles Times* (November 16, 1985). "Aspirin Labels to Warn about Reye Syndrome," *New York Times* (March 8, 1986).

CHAPTER NINE: Triumph and Dissent

179 "This triumphalist account of . . ." "CSM Update: Reye's Syndrome and Aspirin," *British Medical Journal* 292 (1986): 1590.

179 "There is good evidence . . ." Patrick L. Remington, Diane Rowley, Harry McGee, William N. Hall, and Arnold S. Monto, "Decreasing Trends in Reye Syndrome and Aspirin Use in Michigan, 1979 to 1984," *Pediatrics* 77 (1986): 93–98.

180 "By the end of . . ." Michael S. Kramer, "Kids Versus Trees: Reye's Syndrome and Spraying for Spruce Budworm in New Brunswick," *Journal of Clinical Epidemiology* 62 (2009): 578.

181 "A critical part of . . ." Alexander, "Obituary," 48. Altman, "Tale of Triumph," 8.

181 "Likewise, the physicians – often . . ." "Reye's Syndrome: Dr. William Schubert—1976," http://www.youtube.com/watch?v=Fg5pUJdCbRk (accessed December 26, 2013).

181 "All of the officers . . ." Pendergrast, *Inside the Outbreaks*, xiv.

182 "Admiration for the public . . ." *1974–2009, National Reye's Syndrome Foundation* (Bryan, OH: National Reye's Syndrome Foundation, 2009).

183 "The physicians who were . . ." "Reye's Syndrome: Dr. William Schubert—1976," http://www.youtube.com/watch?v=Fg5pUJdCbRk (accessed December 26, 2013).

183 "The height of the . . ." Ermias Belay, Joseph Bresee, Robert C. Holman, Ali S. Khan, Abtin Shahriari, and Lawrence Schonberger, "Reye's Syndrome in the United States from 1981 Through 1997," *New England Journal of Medicine* 340 (1999): 1377–1382.

184 "The entire discussion section . . ." Belay, Bresee,. Holman, Khan, Shahriari, and Schonberger, "Reye's Syndrome in the United States from 1981 Through 1997," 1380–81.

185 "The retrospective study of . . ." Arnold S. Monto, "The Disappearance of Reye's Syndrome—a Public Health Triumph," *The New England Journal of Medicine* 340 (1999): 1423–1424.

186 "I began writing this . . ." Lawrence K. Altman, "Tale of Triumph on Every Aspirin Bottle," *New York Times* (May 11, 1999).

187 "Orlowski's first publication on . . ." James P. Orlowski, Johann H. Johannsson, and Nancy G. Ellis, "Encephalopathy and Fatty Metamorphosis of the Liver Associated with Cold-Agglutinin Autoimmune Hemolytic Anemia," *The Journal of Pediatrics* 4 (1979): 569–575.

187 "Both the symptoms and . . ." Orlowski, Johannsson, and Ellis, "Encephalopathy and Fatty Metamorphosis of the Liver Associated with Cold-Agglutinin Autoimmune Hemolytic Anemia," 573–574. John F. S. Crocker and Philip C. Bagnell, "Reye's Syndrome: A Clinical Review," *Canadian Medical Association Journal* 124 (1981): 375–382.

189 "The first published statement . . ." Boutros, Esfandiari, Orlowski, and Smith, "Reye's Syndrome," 539–552. James P. Orlowski, "Mannitol Crosses the Blood-Brain Barrier in Reye's Syndrome," *Cleveland Clinic Quarterly* 49 (1982): 119–125. James P. Orlowski, "Pediatric Cerebral Resuscitation," *Cleveland Clinic Quarterly* 50 (1983): 317–321. Thomas J. Halpin, Francis J. Holtzhauer, Robert J. Campbell, Lois J. Hall, Adolfo Correa-Villaseñor, Richard Lanese, Janet Rice, and Eugene S. Hurwitz, "Reye's Syndrome and Medication Use," *Journal of the American Medical Association* 248 (1982): 687–691.

189 "Orlowski explained in his . . ." James P. Orlowski, "Aspirin and Reye's Syndrome," *Journal of the American Medical Association* 249 (1983): 3177.

189 "The authors of the . . ." Thomas J. Halpin, Francis J. Holtzhauer, Robert J. Campbell, Lois J. Hall, Adolfo Correa-Villaseñor, Richard Lanese, Janet Rice, and Eugene S. Hurwitz, "Aspirin and Reye's Syndrome," *Journal of the American Medical Association* 249 (1983): 3177. The errata were published in the *New England Journal of Medicine* 249 (1983): 354.

190 "The following year, Orlowski . . ." Philip K. Lichtenstein, James E. Heubi, Cynthia C. Daugherty, Michael K. Farrell, Ronald J. Sokol, Robert J. Rothbaum, Frederick J. Suchy, and William F. Balistreri, "Grade I Reye's Syndrome: A Frequent Cause of Vomiting and Liver Dysfunction after Varicella and Upper-Respiratory-Tract Infection," *New England Journal of Medicine* 309 (1983): 133–139. James P. Orlowski, "Grade I Reye's Syndrome," *New England Journal of Medicine* 310 (1984): 128. Phillip K. Lichtenstein and James E. Heubi, "Grade I Reye's Syndrome," *New England Journal of Medicine* 310 (1984): 129.

190 “That same year — 1984 . . .” James P. Orlowksi, “Aspirin and Reye’s Syndrome: How Strong an Association?” *Postgraduate Medicine* 75 (1984): 47–54. Harry McGee, personal communication, April 8, 2014.

191 “Orlowski published his most . . .” James P. Orlowski, Johnathan Billis, and Henry A. Kilham, “A Catch in the Reye,” *Pediatrics* 80 (1987): 638–642.

192 “Several critical letters followed . . .” Harry B. McGee and Dean Sienko, “A Catch in the Reye,” *Pediatrics* 82 (1988): 390–391. James P. Orlowski, “A Catch in the Reye,” *Pediatrics* 82 (1988): 391. Susan M. Hall, “A Catch in ‘A Catch in the Reye,’” *Pediatrics* 82 (1988): 392–394. Patrick L. Remington and Kevin Sullivan, “A Catch in the Reye,” *Pediatrics* 82 (1988): 676–677. Harry McGee, personal communication, April 8, 2014.

193 “Orlowski’s views on Reye’s . . .” James P. Orlowski, “Whatever Happened to Reye’s Syndrome? Did It Ever Really Exist?” *Critical Care Medicine* 27 (1999): 1582–1587.

193 “Three years later, in . . .” James P. Orlowski, Usama A. Hanhan, and Mariano R. Fialllos, “Is Aspirin a Cause of Reye’s Syndrome?” *Drug Safety* 25 (2002): 225–231.

194 “In many ways, Orlowski’s . . .” Mortimer, “Reye’s Syndrome, Salicylates, Epidemiology, and Public Health,” 1941. A. P. Mowat, “Reye’s Syndrome: 20 Years On,” *British Medical Journal* 286 (1983): 1999–2001. John T. Wilson and R. Don Brown, “Reye Syndrome and Aspirin Use: The Role of Prodromal Illness Severity in the Assessment of Relative Risk,” *Pediatrics* 69 (1982): 822.

195 “For Orlowski to remain . . .” Orlowski, Gillis, and Kilham, “A Catch in the Reye,” *Pediatrics* 80 (1987): 642. Subcommittee on Natural Resources, Agriculture Research, and Environment of the Committee on Science and Technology, “Reye’s Syndrome,” 117–118.

195 “At the hearing, Orlowski . . .” James P. Orlowski, “Aspirin and Reye’s Syndrome,” *Journal of the American Medical Association* 249 (1983): 3177. Subcommittee on Natural Resources, Agriculture Research, and Environment of the Committee on Science and Technology, “Reye’s Syndrome,” 120–121.

CHAPTER TEN: The Politics of Public Health

199 "But, even if I . . ." Belay, Bresee, Holman, Khan, Shahriari, and Schonberger, "Reye's Syndrome in the United States from 1981 through 1997," 1377.

200 "After all my research . . ." The term "Reye's syndrome" appeared for the first time in May 1965. See H. Giles, "Encephalopathy and Fatty Degeneration of the Viscera," *Lancet* 1 (1965): 1075. Two months later, in July 1965, two more articles used the term in two additional journals, which suggested it was in common use by then. See Martin Randolph, Ramon Kranwinkel, Ronald Johnson, Nelson Gelfman, "Encephalopathy, Hepatitis and Fat Accumulation in Viscera," *American Journal of Diseases of Children* 109 (1965): 95–99 and Gerald S. Golden and David Duffell, "Encephalopathy and Fatty Change in the Liver and Kidney," *Pediatrics* 36 (1965): 67–74. Examples of authors who used the term "Reye-Johnson syndrome include Chaves-Carballo, Ellefson, and Gomez, "An Aflatoxin in the Liver of a Patient," 48–50. Joan L. Venes, Bennett A. Shaywitz, and Dennis D. Spencer, "Management of Severe Cerebral Edema in the Metabolic Encephalopathy of Reye-Johnson Syndrome," *Journal of Neurosurgery* 48 (1978): 903–915. E. S. Kang, K. S. Schwenzer, H. P. Wall, J. T. Jabbour, R. Shade, J. T. Crofton, and L. Share, "Urea, Altered Renal Function, and Vasopressin in Reye-Johnson Syndrome," *Biochemical Medicine* 27 (1982): 121–134. For an example of a publications from researchers associated with the Mayo Clinic who referred to the ailment as "Reye-Johnson syndrome," see E. Chaves–Carballo, R. D. Ellefson, and M. R. Gomez, "Hepatic Lipids in Reye-Johnson Syndrome and in Acute Encephalopathy without Fatty Liver," *Mayo Clinic Proceedings* 51 (1976): 770–776. George M. Johnson, "Reye's Syndrome," *American Journal of Diseases of Children* 120 (1970): 89.

201 "Certainly Johnson's inability to . . ." Subcommittee on Natural Resources, Agriculture Research, and Environment of the Committee on Science and Technology, "Reye's Syndrome," 21–22. George Magnus Johnson, "Reye's Syndrome and Salicylates," *New England Journal of Medicine* 314 (1986): 921. Johnson, "Reye's Syndrome," *New England Journal of Medicine* 341 (1999): 846.

202 "The tension between physicans . . ." Spitzer, Hattwick, Hurwitz, Kramer, Kupper, Larke, Pollack, Shank, Seliske, "Report of the New Brunswick Task Force on the Environment and Reye's Syndrome," *Clinical Investigative Medicine* 5 (1982): 203e14.

203 "In Canada, the epidemiologists' . . ." In Ohio, the published rate was 1.04 cases per 100,000 persons, and in Michigan it was estimated that Reye's syndrome appeared in between 30.8 and 57.8 cases of influenza B. See John Z. Sullivan-Bolyai, James S. Marks, Deane Johnson, David B. Nelson, Frank Holtzhauer, Frank Bright, Taylor Kramer, and Thomas J. Halpin, "Reye Syndrome in Ohio, 1973–1977," *American Journal of Epidemiology* 112 (1980): 629–638 and Lawrence Corey, Robert, J. Rubin, Theodore R. Thompson, Gary R. Noble, Edward Cassidy, Michael A. W. Hattwick, Michael B. Gregg, and Donald Eddins, "Influenza B-Associated Reye's Syndrome Incidence in Michigan and Potential for Prevention," *Journal of Infectious Diseases* 135 (1977): 398–407. Kramer, "Kids Versus Trees," 580. Here is the report they produced: Spitzer WO, Hattwick MA, Hurwitz E, Kramer M, Kupper L, Larke RPB, et al. Report of the New Brunswick Task Force on the environment and Reye's syndrome. *Clinical Investigative Medicine* 5 (1982): 203e14.

204 "In 1983, after the . . ." Thomas H. Weller, "Varicella and Herpes Zoster: Changing Concepts of the Natural History, Control, and Importance of a Not-So-Benign Virus (Second of Two Parts)," *New England Journal of Medicine* 309 (1983): 1434–1440. Baral, "Varicella and Herpes Zoster," 329.

204 "The suggestion that Mortimer . . ." Committee on Infectious Diseases, "Aspirin and Reye Syndrome," *Pediatrics* 69 (1982): 810–812. Edward A. Mortimer, Jr., "Reye's Syndrome, Salicylates, Epidemiology, and Public Health Policy," *Journal of the American Medical Association* 257 (1987): 1941. Eugene S. Hurwitz and Edward A. Mortimer, Jr., "A Catch in the Reye is Awry," *Cleveland Journal of Medicine* 57 (1990): 318–319.

205 "Since the turn of . . ." Examples of books that mention the history of Reye's syndrome in the context of the politicization of science include Thomas O. McGarity and Wendy Elizabeth Wagner, *Bending Science: How Special Interests Corrupt Public Health Research*; Oreskes and Conway, *Merchants of Doubt*; and Michaels, *Doubt is Their Product*.

205 "Casting the history of . . ." Charles C. Mann and Mark L. Plummer, *The Aspirin Wars: Money, Medicine, and 100 Years of Rampant Competition* (Boston: Harvard Business School Press, 1991).

206 "In the late 1970s . . ." Mann and Plummer, *The Aspirin Wars*, 227–228. Mann and Plummer cite "Total Analgesic Market Sales and Share Trend Report, Exhibit 5, W. T. Eldridge, Affidavit in Opposition to Motion to Strike or Sever, July 8, 1986, *American Home Products* v. *Johnson & Johnson* (2), Docket.

207 "In the first of . . ." Douglas Martin, "William Conner, Judge Expert in Patent Law, Dies at 89," *New York Times* (July 19, 2009). Mann and Plummer, *The Aspirin Wars*, 229. Bruce Horovitz, "Victory for Advil: Tylenol Claims Misled Public, N.Y. Judge Says," *Los Angeles Times* (February 28, 1987).

208 "At the same time . . ." Andrew H. Malcolm, "Tylenol Maker Recalls Capsules after Strychnine Incident in West," *New York Times* (October 6, 1982). Dan Fletcher, "A Brief History of the Tylenol Poisonings," *Time* (February 9, 1982). Mann and Plummer, *The Aspirin Wars*, 217–219.

208 "By the 1990s, Tylenol..." Arthur F. Varner, William W. Busse, and Robert F. Lemanske, Jr., "Hypothesis: Decreased Use of Pediatric Aspirin has Contributed to the Increasing Prevalence of Childhood Asthma," *Annals of Allergy, Asthma, & Immunology* 81 (1998): 347–351. Christie Aschwanden, "Studies Suggest an Acetaminophen-Asthma Link," *New York Times* (December 19, 2011).

209 "In the fall of..." John T. McBride, "The Association of Acetaminophen and Asthma Prevalence and Severity," *Pediatrics* 128 (2011): 1181–1185. C. C. Johnson and D. R. Ownby, "Have the Efforts to Prevent Aspirin-Related Reye's Syndrome Fuelled an Increase in Asthma?" *Clinical & Experimental Allergy* 41 (2011): 296–298.

Index

Bellevue Literary Press is devoted to publishing literary fiction and nonfiction at the intersection of the arts and sciences because we believe that science and the humanities are natural companions for understanding the human experience. With each book we publish, our goal is to foster a rich, interdisciplinary dialogue that will forge new tools for thinking and engaging with the world.

To support our press and its mission, and for our full catalogue of published titles, please visit us at blpress.org.

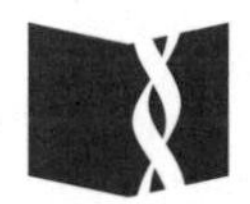

Bellevue Literary Press
New York